THE BOOK ON PALO

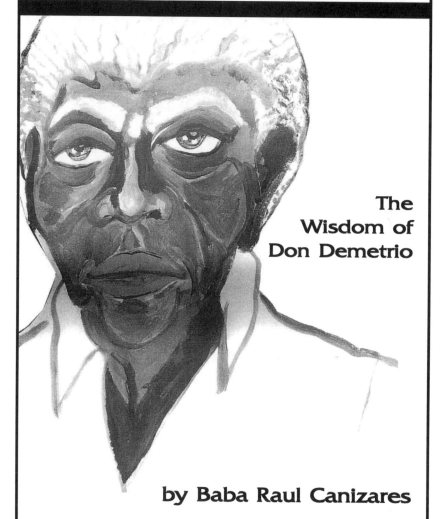

The
Wisdom of
Don Demetrio

by Baba Raul Canizares

ORIGINAL PUBLICATIONS

THE BOOK ON PALO

By Baba Raul Canizares

© ORIGINAL PUBLICATIONS 2002

ISBN: 0-942272-66-8

FIRST EDITION
First Printing 2002

Interior illustrations by Raul Canizares

Original Publications
P.O. Box 236
Old Bethpage, New York 11804-0236
(516) 454-6809

Printed in the United States of America

ACKNOWLEDGMENT

Although It is not my custom to feature an acknowledgment page in my books, I simply had to have one in this one. There are so many people that contribute to any endeavor such as a book that reflects the teachings one has accumulated over the years, that an honest acknowledgment section would be as thick as the book itself. In the case of **THE BOOK ON PALO**, however, not to mention Marc Benezra would be tantamount to dishonesty.

The reason why a Palo book of this magnitude has never been attempted is because the nature of Palo itself is an editor's nightmare. Palo depends on ideograms, highly idiosyncratic use of KiKongo, and specific chants called mambos to communicate its message. Even the great Lydia Cabrera only scratched the surface in her volumes dedicated to Palo. Yet, as demonstrated here, a fairly complete book on Palo was possible, and we have done it. By "we" I mean Marc Benezra and I (with the invaluable help of Milton Benezra, who gave the book its final touches). More than any other book I've worked on before, this is a collaborative effort. I'm sure Marc has invested as many hours editing as I have writing it. The result is a work I am proud to call my own.

I first proposed the Book on Palo to Marc's Father, Milton, back in 1992, Marc and I started working on it in 1999, and we finished it in August, 2002. Looking over it, I see that it really needed such detailed care, for I hope all who read it will feel the effort and professionalism, not to mention love and care, that went into it. I honestly don't think this book would have its present scope without Marc Benezra's effort. Thanks seems somehow redundant, but it will have to do.

INTRODUCTION

Palo is one of four main African-derived religions still practiced in Cuba, the other three are *Santeria, Abakuá, and Arará.* The religion developed among practitioners of a form of necromancy called *Nganga* which is still widely found in various parts of the west coast of Central Africa. "Nganga" refers both to the practice and to its priests. In Cuba, the practitioners of Nganga were mostly of KiKongo and BaKongo stock. Highly utilitarian and syncretistic even in Africa, Palo, as the practice of Nganga came to be known in Cuba, added to the Congo, Yoruba, Arab, and Dahomean mix it brought from Africa, popular Roman Catholicism, Kardecian Spiritism, and elements of Freemasonry in Cuba.

Palo has four branches; *Palo Briyumba, Palo Monte, Palo Mayombe,* and *Palo Kimbisa.* Palo Briyumba has the most African retentions. Palo Monte is mostly identified with goodness, while Palo Mayombe is thought to be "evil." Palo Kimbisa is the most Christianized and Masonic of the Palo sects.

The focus of this book is on Palo Monte as taught by Demetrio Gomez Camposanto Medianoche (1874-1968). Guanabacoa, the town Demetrio calls home, is on the outskirts of Havana and is famous for keeping African traditions alive. I was initiated into Palo by Demetrio when I was a small child, he died when I was twelve. His student Paco kept careful notes on Demetrio's wisdom. After Demetrio's death, Paco went on to become a priest of Ifá, abandoning the practice of Palo. Before his own death in 1985, Paco generously shared his invaluable notes on Demetrio with me.

Beginning in chapter one, it will be Demetrio's voice you will hear, channeled through mine. May God Almighty Zambia bless all our efforts.

Baba Raul Canizares
founder, Orisha Consciousness Movement,
Tata, Munanzo Tiembla Tierra,
New York, NY, 6/06/99

CHAPTER I

WHAT IS PALO MONTE?

My Christian name is Demetrio Gomez, both of my parents, Jose Herrera and Francisquilla Perez, were born in Angola. They were brought to Cuba as slaves. It was in Cuba that they met while serving the same master, a relatively poor Spaniard named Don Triburcio Perez. Don Triburcio had a small farm in Guanabacoa where he raised pigs. He only owned three slaves; his wife and children used to labor right alongside them, so there was a feeling among the slaves of belonging to a family rather than being owned by slavemasters.

Shortly after I was born a strange sickness killed off most of Don Triburcio's pigs and he faced losing his property. In order to raise money, he was forced to sell my father to a wealthy aristocrat named Demetrio Gumersindo Gomez Chaviano, who paid an incredibly high price for him. Back in Africa, my father had been a feared Nganga. Don Demetrio, who knew the power of African magic, had heard of my father's gifts as a practitioner. Thinking my father's talents were being wasted raising pigs, as soon as he brought his new slave to his property he encouraged him to set up shop as a Palero, as Ngangas were called in Cuba. My father would provide Don Demetrio as well as the numerous slaves and free men who worked the sugar cane plantation with his special kind of

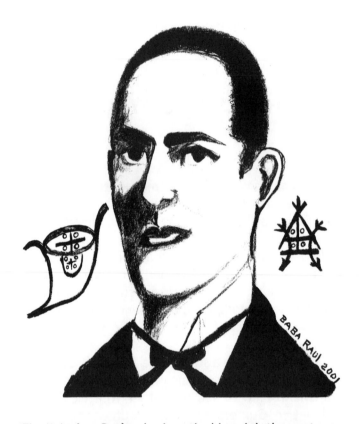

(Fig. 1) **Andres Petit,** *charismatic, bi-racial, thaumaturge who in the mid-1800's founded the Kimbisa faction of Palo religion. He also led a group of Abakuá religionists. Petit opened African spiritualities in Cuba to whites by initiating them as priests.*

service. In less than a year, Don Demetrio came to view my father as his spiritual mentor and principal problem-solver.

Andres Petit, a free man of color who befriended both Don Demetrio and my father was another powerful practitioner of Palo. Petit, an elegant, impeccably dressed, and charismatic man who was greatly admired by most, convinced my father to initiate Don Demetrio into the mysteries of Palo in exchange for his freedom. Petit had his detractors and was criticized by other blacks for "selling out the secrets of African magic" to whites. In reality, initiating whites into African magical systems was a brilliant act of empowerment for the initiators, since it virtually put the white initiates in the subservient position of neophytes in relation to their black teachers.

Don Triburcio absolutely refused to sell my mother to Don Demetrio. Triburcio's children considered their nana as much a part of their family as Don Triburcio's wife, Doña Emilia. My father was allowed to visit my mother as often as he could. I was baptized in the Catholic Church when I was about one and a half. Don Demetrio and his wife, Doña Petra, became my Catholic god-parents. Eventually Don Triburcio agreed to let me move in with my father. By the time Don Triburcio died in 1880 slavery had been abolished in Cuba. He left my mother a comfortable cottage in a small plot of land near his farm in Guanabacoa. At last my family was reunited. It was in that cottage, where I still live, that my father and other men from the "old Country," as Africa was called, taught me how to be a Palero. Old J.S. Baró, a former slave from the Belgian Congo, taught me about Palo Mayombe, Andres Petit initiated me into Palo Kimbisa, yet it was my father's intimate knowledge of Palo Monte that most deeply affected me.

Palo Monte is my TRUTH. It is also the truth for thousands of others. I would never say that Palo is "the TRUTH." No one religion should claim to be the sole repository of the TRUTH. I reject no religion except those that routinely practice coercion, exploitation, and/or dishonesty. The teachings I leave behind are intended for

5

those who would benefit from the practice of Palo Monte. Palo is not for everyone. In my sixty years as a Palero I have rejected ten times as many people as I have accepted for initiation. Those who need to be here will find their way. Palo Monte teaches trust in God, belief in destiny, and respect for the forces that move the Universe. These forces can take surprising forms and can manifest themselves in unusual and unexpected manners. In a world steeped in despair, any path that brings solace and spiritual fortitude should be allowed to flourish. The practice of Palo Monte engenders a particular form of spiritual strength, a gutsy, down-in-your-groin, earthy power that some people need to experience as their souls travel on the way to the Final Cause.

Palo Monte, Vodou, and Macumba have much in common. Although what I know of Brazilian Macumba is mostly second hand, I have spent months at a time in Haiti studying Petro Vodou and I can tell you that it is similar enough to Palo Monte for both religions to be considered branches of the same tree. The first lesson for the would-be Palero is that this religion is as valid as Christianity, Islam, or Buddhism. To fully understand African traditional religions, the outsider who seeks shelter in one of them, such as Palo Monte, has to leave behind pre-conceived ideas about the wild, sensual, horrific "voodoo" cults depicted in Hollywood films. Such grotesque imagery has two principal historical precedents: the overwrought tourist shows put on in Haiti for the benefit of thrill-seeking foreigners, and the deliberately wild dances orchestrated on Congo Square and other places in New Orleans during the last half of the 19th century. These spectacles were put on by a series of Voodoo queens, the most notable being Marie Laveau, for the benefit of high-paying white onlookers. Although Madame Laveau was undoubtedly a powerful practitioner, she was also a sharp business-woman who knew how to put on a lucrative show. The religious aspects of Palo, Macumba, and Vodou, however, have nothing to do with these aberrations. In a concise manner, I'll describe in the following notes the basics of Palo Monte, including its deities, initiatory rituals and ceremonies, as well as the relationship between Palo deities, Yoruba orishas, and Catholic saints. I'll also provide a glossary of Palo terms consisting of creolized KiKongo, and, most importantly, a compilation of some of the most popular and effective mambos. The Palo invocations known as mambos are of supreme importance in calling forth the spiritual forces that we work with; therefore, learning these mambos is essential to a Palero's growth.

We Paleros do not proselytize, since we do not believe that ours is the only way. *"Many are the roads that lead to Heaven,"* states one of our proverbs. Although some anthropologists have criticized us for being syncretistic, mixing elements of many other paths, they fail to realize that this could also be said of any other religion. Palo is as ancient as any other faith. Adapting and changing is just part of our tradition, a way of surviving. Palo has all the hallmarks of a valid religion, including a well-defined set of ethics and morals which teach respect for human life, the sharing of wealth with those who are less fortunate, and belief in a supreme god called ZAMBIA, as well as in his helpers, the NKISIS, also commonly called "orishas" (a term we borrowed from our Yoruba neighbors back in Africa) . We also have what I call a "natural priesthood" consisting of men and women who have been chosen by the wise spirits and the orishas to be set apart as teachers, herbalists, counselors, and messengers between the world of the seen and of the unseen. Palo priests and priestesses, therefore, must become proficient in the art of communicating with enlightened disencarnate intelligences we call "pure essences" or "pure spirits". We also believe that sometimes backward, evil essences can be manipulated and used by the Palero. If the Palero is a practitioner of mostly beneficial magic, the evil spirit may be helped to evolve into a good spirit. An unscrupulous Palero may also use these unfortunate souls for his own benefit without caring for the spiritual development of the backward spirits. The evildoer will then have to face the consequences of his actions at some future point, and the impure essence that had been misused by the Palero may encounter a good teacher in the future who will help him or her develop, so in God's eyes the whole evil/good dichotomy is just a play leading to eventual order and balance. All Paleros believe that, ultimately, good will triumph over evil.

Palo Monte teaches that all that exists was created by Zambia-God. He created good as well as evil—the reasons why he did this are ultimately unknown to us in the material plane, although theologians and philosophers may argue about it till the cows come home. Pure spirits incarnate in the material world in order to live out their destiny here for as long as it is necessary in order to learn what can only be learned in the material plane, in order to advance to the realm of the spirits (also called the realm of the essences) or to the realm of Truth, from which no reincarnation is necessary.

The ideographs, painted "signatures", recited chants, performed invocations, and conducted seances designed to communicate with the pure spirits form the core of the practice of Palo Monte. We who are initiated in the path of Palo Monte are called "Paleros." Although some may find this appellation humorous ("Palero" means "user of sticks"), we find no fault with this name and accept it with dignity and honor. In my own house (congregation) we are under the protection of *Centella Ndoki,* the goddess of lightning, and are committed to seeking out that which is beneficial and just for all members. We maintain constant communication with enlightened essences in order to receive their guidance, wisdom, and beneficent care for all who come under the protection of this house (munanzo) under the divine care of Centella Ndoki. Our religion consists in belief in a high God whom we praise, a number of demigods who we actively worship and interact with, the pure spirits we constantly work with, a hierarchical priesthood, a body of believers, temples, altars, and traditional rituals passed on from generation to generation by way of our ancestors.

Most of my godchildren are simple, hardworking folk. Many have been victimized by systems not friendly to the poor and disenfranchised. Many of these people have been turned away by conventional sources of support and have come to view our spirits and deities are their last hope for justice. Palo Monte is a utilitarian and practical religion, more concerned with the here and now than with the hereafter. We recognize GOD (ZAMBIA) as the highest being. Borrowing a Yoruba word, in our munanzo we call the demigods

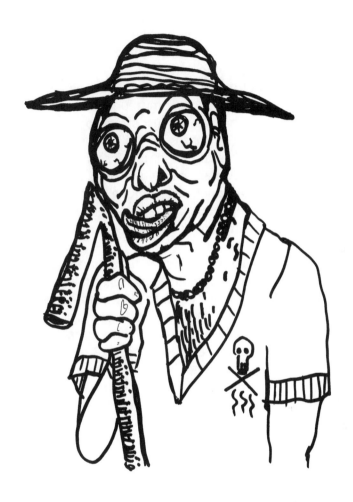

(Fig.2) **Lugambé:** *An old trickster spirit often called "demonic" in Palo treatises. He was Demetrio Gomez's main spirit guide.*

"orishas" interchangeably with "nkisis," which is the more traditional KiKongo term. The orishas have power over everything that happens, both good and evil. Unlike Santeria, which does not teach that there exists an eternal duality of good vs. evil, we Paleros believe that there is a clear and long-standing battle between absolute good and absolute evil, the tension between the two being the energy that propels existence. In my munanzo, called MUNANZO CENTELLA NDOKI, I teach that we must strive to do good. We are committed to fighting the forces of evil. Our temple here in Guanabacoa is simple. There is a major *"prenda"* (cauldron) for worship and another one we actually work with. The major prenda is dedicated to Centella Ndoki, the working prenda, inhabited by an old trickster spirit called Lungambé (see Fig. 2), is used in all of the temple's dealings with the dead—the essences.

Our hierarchical structure is simple. The head of the temple is called the "Tata Nganga" (a female would be the Nana Nganga). In Spanish, our members call the Tata "Padrino," which means Godfather. Anyone seeking membership in our munanzo and who is ultimately accepted by the Tata must undergo the "Purification and Acceptance" initiation, also known as "Presentation to the Nganga." At this stage the neophyte becomes a member of the munanzo and is called "ahijado" or "ahijada" (godson or goddaughter). Later on, the neophyte may receive further instructions preparing him or her for further development. The next step after presentation is the SCRATCHING ceremony. After a period of time where the neophyte and the godfather have had a chance to assess each other for a minimum of three months, the neophyte may request that the godfather ask the orishas and the spirits if the neophyte is ready to be offered a more advanced initiation. Although everyone can benefit from being presented to the Nganga, not many are called to go deeper than that. If a godchild is accepted for scratching, he or she receives certain ceremonial scratches on the skin and is given certain information not available to non-scratched people. This information has to do with sacred formulas and practices that empower the newly scratched Palero. After a year and seven days of having been scratched, a godchild may request to be given his/her own cauldron. The cauldron *(prenda, nganga)* is a miniature universe containing at least 21 sticks *(palos, where the religion gets its name)* and other secret ingredients which imbue it with enormous power. Paleros are supposed to concentrate on developing their particular talents, such as ritual expert, healer, herbalist, exorcist, drummer, singer, or diviner. He or she will develop these attributes through the grace *(ashé)* of his elders.

Every godchild has an obligation to aid his godfather in whatever the godchild can. This should include offering help in maintaining the temple and the altars themselves extremely clean and filled with flowers and sweet-smelling colognes. All members of the house should learn how to divine using four pieces of coconut or four shells (chomolongos). The most common and accepted form of divination in Palo is to communicate directly with the essences while these essences possess Palo priests, taking over their senses and speaking through them. My father taught me that when orishas possess Paleros, these are really avatars of the orishas, not the totality of those great spirits—unless the Palero happens to also be a Santero, in which case and under the right circumstances, the archetypal orishas may possess them. Paradoxically, however, when a Palero communicates with an avatar, he is actually communicating with the great spirits, because these avatars are part of those great beings as much as a drop of coffee that spills out of a cup is of the same substance as the greater amount that remains inside the cup. Some Paleros feel that the best method of communicating with the orishas is to use the *diloggun* or cowry shells method of divination, since it is said that the primal force of the orishas speak through these sixteen shells. Another advantage of using shells rather than possession as a way of communicating with the orishas is that the priest does not lose his consciousness to the orisha, as it happens during possession. It also requires less effort to cast the shells than to become possessed.

During the time of persecution, which intermittently lasted well into the middle of the present century, Paleros were forced to hide

11

their deities under the guise of Catholic saints. Back in Africa, Ngangas had already developed a correspondence between their deities and those of the Yoruba pantheon. What follows is a list of our most popular deities, their Catholic counterparts and their Yoruba names.

PALO MONTE	CATHOLIC	YORUBA / SANTERIA
Nkisis, Kimpungulu	saints, celestial court	orishas
Zambia, Nsambi Mpungu	God Almighty	Olodumare
Nkuyo, Lucero	Child of Prague, St. Anthony, Lonely Soul	Eshu, Elegbara
Mama Kengue, Tiembla-Tierra	Our Lady of Mercy, Jesus	Obatalá, Oshanlá
Nsasi, Siete Rayos	St. Barbara	Shangó
Kalunga, Balaunde Madre de Agua	O.L. of Regla	Yemayá, Olokun
Mama Shola	O.L. of Charity	Oshún
Kubayende, Pata en Llaga	St. Lazarus	Babalú Aiyé, Shakpana
Zarabanda	St. Peter, St. John the Baptist	Ogún
Mariwanga, Centella Ndoki	St. Therese	Oyá
Watariamba, Vence Batallas, Busca Rastros	St. Norbert	Oshosi

PALO MONTE	CATHOLIC	YORUBA / SANTERIA
Tata Funde, Cuatro Vientos, Daday	St. Francis of Assisi	Orunmila, Ifá
Musilango	St. Isidore	Orishaoko
Burufinda, Ngurufinda	St. Joseph	Osanyin, Osain
Mama Canata	O.L. of Mount Carmel	Nana Bukuu
Brazo Fuerte	St. Christopher	Aganju

In Cuba the language we use in our ceremonies is called "Palo" or "Bantu." It derives mainly from KiKongo, with plenty of creolized Spanish and some Yoruba thrown in for good measure. When sacrificing animals, we always call them by their Palo names, thus a rooster is called *ensuso*, a sheep *enkonde,* a goat *meme,* the rum we spray from our mouths in a ceremonial fashion *malafo*, the sacrificial knife *embele-koto*, gunpowder *fula,* water *lanso,* gourd dish *tie tie*, machete *embele*, the razor blade we use to scratch neophytes *gele-samba*, the cigar we use to offer our spirits blessed smoke *ensunga,* and incense is *maba-guindango*. Ahead a more extensive glossary will be provided.

The first sign of initiation the neophyte receives after the purification/presentation ceremony is the "necklace." Wearing this necklace indicates that the person is a member of the munanzo and is entitled to the godfather's protection as well as help from all members of the munanzo, including the spirit protectors, who are considered an integral part of the house. Along with the necklace, the neophyte is given a set of rules and guides to follow. Becoming a member of a munanzo carries with it privileges, but also responsibilities. If after getting the necklace the neophyte neglects his/her duties, then he or she may become vulnerable to misfortune, the spirits letting the person know that life is a two-way street: neglect your responsibilities to me, and I'll neglect mine to you, the spirits might say. Every munanzo should take care to celebrate its important feasts, such as its Tata's initiation day and the days of the most important orishas.

Our munanzo is fairly varied, most of our members are hard-working people, although we do have a couple of important political figures and several showbizz luminaries that are faithful Paleros. One of the factors that unites us is our devotion to LUNGAMBÉ, the spirit of our temple's working nganga, who in our house takes the form of a deceptively funny old man who constantly licks his lips. Lungambé, an avatar of Eshu, is Centella Ndoki's messenger. Lungambé's principal spirit helper is Perro Bernardo, who likes to present himself as a not-too-advanced essence who nevertheless "gets the job done." The fact is that Perro Bernardo is very bright, he just enjoys playing down his intelligence. Other spirits we work with are El Hermano Jose, an extremely wise old black man who died in 1915, and Candelo Blanc, also known as Le Flambeau, a Haitian Petro spirit. Pure spirits may not have the answer to all our problems, but they do have the advantage of not being fettered by a material body and of being able to detect lies and fraud. After experiencing a thousand and one adventures with these and many other spirits, I've come to regard them as members of my family, as real and present as my wife or my children. These spirits are our protectors; they deserve all our love, praise, and devotion.

Let me again reiterate why I am instructing those to whom I am dictating these words to make them public after I am gone. As both Palo and Santeria emerge from secrecy and as more and more practitioners are willing to speak up publically, the need for accurate information regarding these formerly closed magical systems will become greater. Another problem that arises with Palo and Santeria's increased visibility is that many dishonest or misinformed people purporting to speak about these faiths will not be presenting an accurate picture. I believe we who have been blessed with a powerful Palo and Santeria foundation must eventually lay aside the veil of secrecy that was used in the past in order to give the world a glimpse of our beautiful traditions. Years ago, participating in African-based religions could cause a person's life or freedom to be taken away. Also, people who practiced African religions were often socially ostracized and persecuted in many subtle ways. Now that such abuses are less frequent, we must lift up our voices and demand that our religions be respected by the world at large.

Coming back to our present task of writing down all that is accurate about Palo, let me say that we consider the coconut sacred; it is an indispensable component of all our rituals. Coconut throwing, more properly called *obi divination*, is an age-old method of communication between humans and spirits. Cowry shell casting, called IBBO, CHOMOLONGO, or COBO in Palo and DILOGGUN in Santeria, grew out of obi divination. Cowry shells are thought to be the "mouths" of the orishas and are considered more accurate than coconuts. In Palo, however, we believe that intense, one-to-one interactions with the pure essences is the highest form of divination.

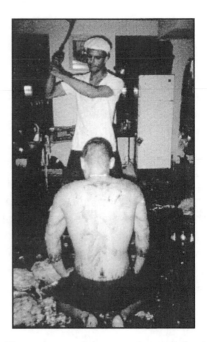

Mayordomo giving newly-scratched neophyte ritual lashing. © Eric Lerner.

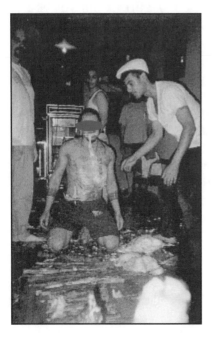

Extremely rare photograph of a "scratching" initiation. In a moment of frenzy, the initiate bites off head of a chicken as Mayordomo Nsambi Kienvence (right) takes care of his new student. © Eric Lerner.

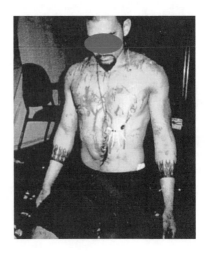

Moment of deep meditation during scratching ceremony. © Eric Lerner.

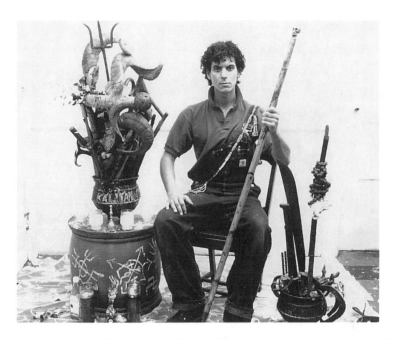

Mayordomo Nsambi Kienvence, a Kimbisa high priest, poses next to two of his *fundamentos,* Centella Ndoki (left) and Sarabanda (right).　　© Alejandro Guzman.

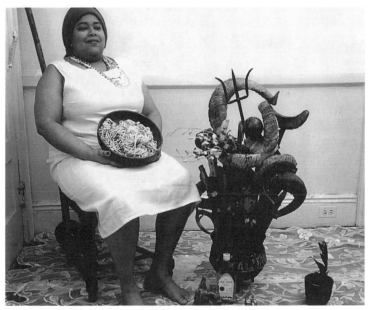

Yayi Luz and Centella Ndoki.　　© Alejandro Guzman.

17

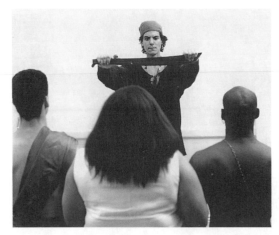

Three neophytes *(ngueyos)* swearing loyalty in front of Sarabanda, God of truth and justice, symbolized by the sabre held by Mayordomo.

© Alejandro Guzman

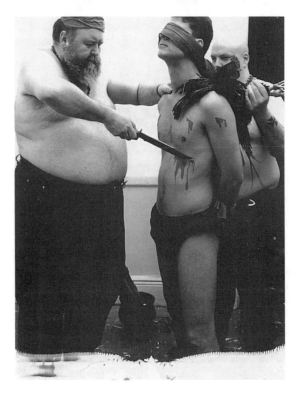

Tata Camposanto Medianoche, A/K/A Baba Raul Canizares "scratching" Moroccan neophyte Adel with the assistance of Italian-American Palero John Andolina, showing Palo's increasingly multi-ethnic composition.

© Alejandro Guzman

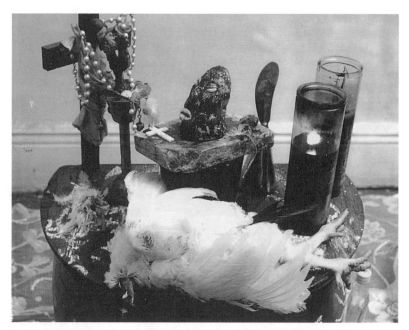

Lucero (center) with chicken sacrifice. © Alejandro Guzman.

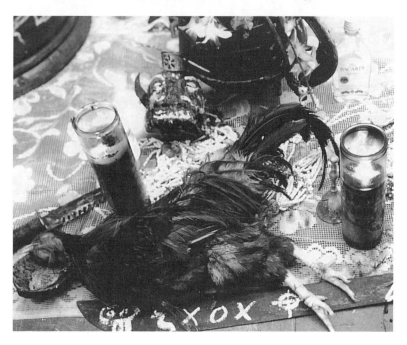

Black rooster sacrifice for Nkuyo. © Alejandro Guzman.

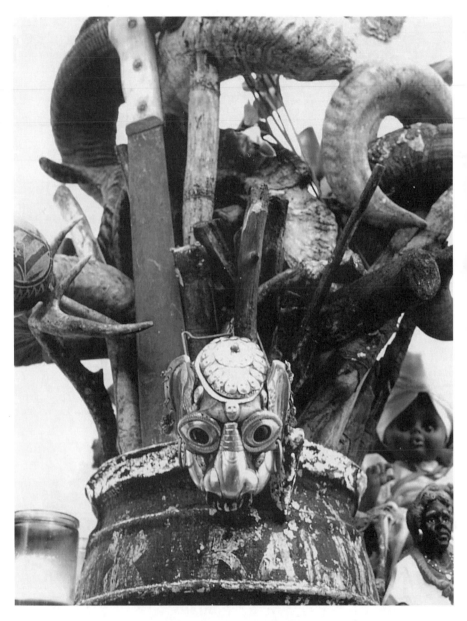

Nganga featuring a silver-inlaid monkey skull from Tibet.   © Alejandro Guzman.

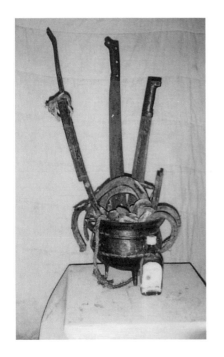

Sarabanda cauldron belonging to Tata Camposanto Medianoche.

© Raul Canizares.

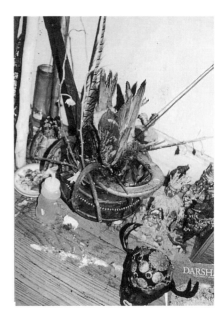

Pigeon sacrifice to Sarabanda cauldron, note horned Nkuyo, forefront.

© Clayton Patterson

21

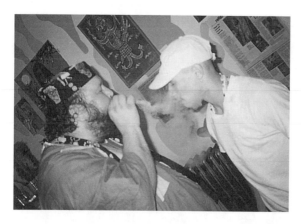

Tata Camposanto Medianoche giving a godson a cigar-smoke cleansing.

© Clayton Patterson

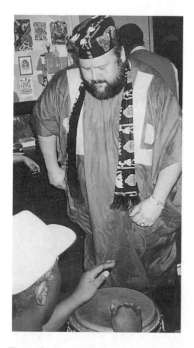

Tata Camposanto Medianoche dancing for the Palo Spirits while legendary percussionist Montego Joe plays the conga.

© Clayton Patterson.

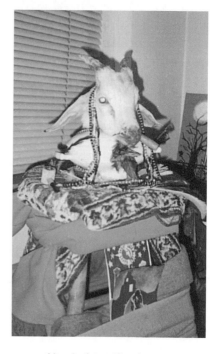

Head of sacrificed goat for Centella Ndoki

© Raul Canizares

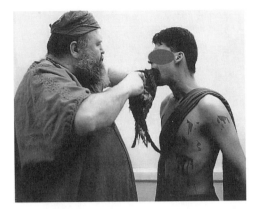

Published for the first time, photo of a neophyte drinking blood from decapitated chicken.

© Alejandro Guzman

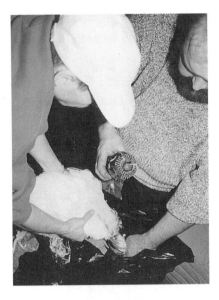

Offering a life to Nkuyo, messenger of the gods.

© Clayton Patterson

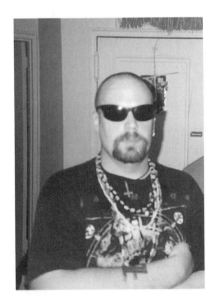

Knowledgeable Italian-American Palero, and Omo Eshu John Andelino from Brooklyn, New York.

© Raul Canizares

23

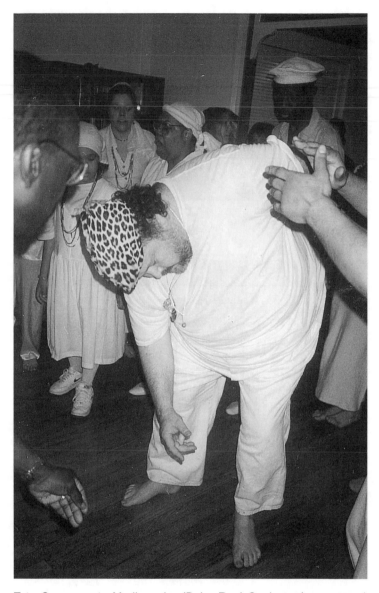

Tata Camposanto Medianoche (Baba Raul Canizares) possessed by Tiembla- Tierra.   © Narayan Ramos

CHAPTER 2

MAKING CHAMBA

Note: most names have been left in Spanish except when I was sure of the English equivalent. Any well-stocked botanica will carry most of the ingredients named in this chapter.
— Raul Canizares

Chamba is the holy liquid of Palo. There are many ways to make chamba. The main ingredients of the chamba we make for multiple uses are:

- Rain water, *particularly that collected during the first rain of the month of May as it settles in the crevices of the silk cotton tree, forming small puddles.*

- River water

- Sea water

- Holy water *from a Catholic or Eastern Orthodox church*

- Palm oil

- Cocoa butter

- Cascarilla or Pembe chalk

- Black pepper kernel

- Eru *(a Nigerian root)*

- Kola nut

- A burning charcoal wrapped in a Malanga leaf

- At least twenty-one of the orisha's herbs

Chamba serves to purify and sanctify stones, necklaces, seashells, amulets, and all kinds of implements used for ritual purposes or to provide protection. The herbs which are to be used in the preparation of chamba should be placed on a straw mat in front of several elders who will chew some of them to imbue the herbs with their ashé (grace). Of those present during the preparation of the chamba, the one with the least amount of time initiated will gather the herbs and, walking on his or her knees as a sign of respect, will hand the herbs over to the elders for chewing. After the elders chew the plants, they will deposit them in clay containers that have been painted in the emblematic colors of each orisha represented. Thus, herbs sacred to Shangó will be deposited in a red container, to Obatalá in a white one, and so on. The elders must have recited the *mo juba prayer* before starting, and must sing to each orisha as he or she works with the different orisha's herbs. The orishas must be sung to in the following order: Lucero, Zarabanda, Oshosi, Tiembla-Tierra, Siete Rayos, Centella Ndoki, Madre de Agua, and Mama Shola, followed by any other orisha that needs to be invoked. In our house, since we have so many Santeros that also practice Palo, we tend to sing Santeria/Yoruba songs when we make chamba. After the sorting-of-the-herbs ceremony, the person with the greatest seniority will lift the straw mat where the herbs had been worked making sure every single bit of herb gets used in the chamba.

Chamba is indispensable in the making of a *ngangulero* (owner of a cauldron). After a scratched member of the munanzo has successfully completed his/her one year and seven days apprenticeship, he or she may ask the Tata for a reading regarding whether he or she is psychologically, spiritually, and physically ready to receive the awesome responsibility of having his/her own nganga (prenda, cauldron). Assuming all goes well and the applicant is accepted for inclusion in the ranks of nganguleros, the tata's assistant, called the *mayordomo* or, if a woman, the *yayi or tikan-tika,* will have to bathe the future ngangulero with chamba seven days in a row. The mayordomo will also make sure his charge drinks three big gulps of chamba each morning. A super-charged chamba will also contain some of the blood of sacrificed animals, as well as some rum. *Aberikolas* (non-initiates) should never view any of the ceremonies discussed so far. After initiation as a ngangulero, the newly-created cauldron-owning priest must be watched closely by the padrino, the mayordomo, or the yayi, for in the week following initiation, his strengths and weakness will be magnified a thousand times; it is the teacher's responsibility to note these strengths and weaknesses in order to guide the new ngangulero through them later in life. Some of the nkisis we have installed in our munanzo include Centella Monte Oscuro, Siete Rayos, Tumba Loma, Vence Batallas, Mariquilla Ndoki, Acaba Mundo, Tranca Vias, and Vira Mundo. These are potent forces. Before we can allow one of our priests to channel one of these spirits, we must be sure he or she can handle it. After one week, we offer the new ngangulero his *Esengue,* a staff made of Iroko wood, while he holds a lit candle which rests on a white plate.

Chamba is also used to feed and invigorate the deities. Lucero's chamba may have three, twenty-one, or one-hundred one different herbs, Tiembla-Tierra takes eight, Siete Rayos six, Centella Ndoki nine, Madre de Agua seven, Mama Shola five, Zarabanda three or seven, Pata en Llaga seventeen, and so on. All herbs must have been duly consecrated as described above. Chamba should be added to any food cooked for the orishas or during feasts. The following are some herbs belonging to the different orishas.

LUCERO: *horsehair, lengua de vaca, grass, wheatgrass, asafetida, itamo real, meloncillo, basil, piñon, yamao.*

TIEMBLA-TIERRA: *bledo de clavo, sauco, encampane, aguinaldo blanco, lillies, higuereta, almond, soursop, marquesa, jagua blanca.*

SIETE RAYOS and **BRAZO FUERTE:** *bledo rojo, atipola, moco de guanajo, baria, platanillo, plantain, banana, sasparilla, china berry, elm, jobo.*

MADRE DE AGUA: *vervain, lechuguilla, indigo, prodigiosa, paraguita, flor de agua, lotus, hyacinth, fern, watercress, hierba buena, purple basil, guasima, boton de oro, yerba de la niña, cucaracha, palo canelo, yerba mora, corazon de paloma.*

ZARABANDA: *lemongrass, pata de gallina, hueso de gallo, mimosa, siempreviva, jericho flower, romerillo, piñon, rompe saraguey, purple basil, ebony.*

CENTELLA NDOKI: *yerba garro, guasimilla, baria, yucca, plum, cabo de hacha, mazorquilla.*

Never put sticks or bark in chamba, only leaves and soft stems. Lucero, Zarabanda, and Oshosi can interchange herbs. So can Madre de Agua and Mama Shola. **Pata en Llaga,** however, must never be mixed in rituals with other orishas, except Nana Bukuu and Afrá. Pata en Llaga's herbs are: *cundiamor, sargazo, pazote, zazafra, ateje, alacrancillo, escoba amarga, piñon, botija, casimón, bejuco ubi, tapa caminos, carabalí la yaya, and téngue.*

We must not forget that the most important ingredient of Chamba is water, the very essence of God's favorite daughter, Oshun, who was incarnated in Angola as a queen named Shola Wanga.

Baths make our members healthy and ready to receive the good vibrations our spirit guides bring. Any prospective member of our munanzo must be given some chamba to drink. He or she will then be bathed in Chamba and taken to a cemetery or a sacred grove where he or she will swear an oath of allegiance to the Tata, the munanzo, and all of its members. Initiations should ideally be carried out outdoors in the wilderness, but placing lots of plants, tree branches, and herbs in a room can substitute for the real thing if circumstances call for it.

CHAPTER 3

IROKO

A plant considered more powerful than all others, including the majestic royal palm, is IROKO, which in Cuba has been identified with the stately silk cotton tree. Paleros sometimes call Iroko *"munanzo mambe"* (house of God). Most Palo Monte houses give Iroko a white chicken offering each month. Iroko is almost never used for evil purposes. The one exception is the making of so-called *ngangas judias* in the Palo Mayombe tradition. The pejorative use of the word "Jew" (judia) to imply evil reflects the anti-Semitic sentiments of the dominant Spanish rulers of nineteenth century Cuba. In reality, most Paleros are not conscious of the offensive nature of the use of this word. I find it interesting that the Jews in my munanzo have never complained about this, even though I've instructed my godchildren not to use the word judia in its negative context. Since all the other houses continue to refer to "prendas judias" and "ngangas judias," I mention this here as a way of teaching what these are. The Mayombero will bury the prenda that will be used for evil purposes under Iroko's shadow for twenty-one days. At that time, a totally black cat will be made to become enraged, when it is then decapitated, its skull and left back tibia being made an integral part of the evil nganga.

TO GET SOMETHING FROM IROKO

To gain Iroko's favor, hard-boil sixteen eggs, removing the shell from each. On the ground on the eastern side of the Iroko tree, draw an equilateral cross using palm oil, then place sixteen pennies and the sixteen peeled eggs, one at a time, over the cross. Place each egg on top of each penny, beginning at the head of the cross down to its feet, then from left to right in the horizontal line. Each time you deposit an egg, say out loud a particular petition—it must be the same petition all sixteen times. At the end, say *"Father Iroko, grant me this boon in twenty-one days, amen."*

TO CALM AN ENEMY

To calm an enemy, boil four eggs until they are hard, peel them, dress them with cocoa butter, almond oil, and Balsamo Tranquilo or oil of cloves. Take the dressed eggs to Iroko, making the offering to Tiembla-Tierra, whose palace is in the top of Iroko. Tiembla Tierra will pacify the most stubborn soul.

Iroko, Father of all trees, gives solace to all who ask. There can be no nganga without Iroko, since its stick is the most important of the twenty-one. When walking by a silk cotton tree, believers must always salute it with respect, saying something like *"good morning, Father Iroko, bless me, your humble servant, with health and peace, and forgive me if I've unwittingly stepped on your holy shadow."*

My father used to call Iroko FUMBE. Spirits called "nfumbi" live in Iroko, where Paleros feed them periodically. These Eshu-like spirits, similar also to the *gede* of Vodou, are offered candy on a brand-new plate. The Palero will write his *firma* (personal ideograph or sigyll) on the ground by the part of the tree's trunk that faces east. Along with the candy, the nfumbi are given four peeled hard-boiled eggs, four clear glasses filled with water, coffee, a lit cigar, and some rum. When a vulture rests on one of Iroko's branches, we Paleros believe it is a sign of Oshun Ibu Kole's favor. This crone aspect of the goddess of sensuality and riches is called Kana-Kana in Palo. The following mambo to Iroko is to be sung after sunset :

Mambo to Iroko
Sanda Narbe
Sanda nkinia naribe
Sanda fumadaga
Ndinga nkusi
Ndiga mundo
Pangualan boco
Medio tango
Malembe Ngusi
Malembe mpolo
Kindiambo kilienso
Guatuka ngusi

Iroko is a natural temple. It is there that we bury our ngangas, our cauldrons, in order to imbue them with enormous power. In places where there are no silk cotton trees, Paleros will travel to places that have them if they are serious about obtaining the greatest amount of power. There are many Iroko trees in the Southern United States. The Seminole Indians worshipped Iroko under the name *"kapok."* Paleros work with Iroko in many different ways. Its trunk is used in tieing down spells; Iroko's shadow serves as a resting place for many spirits that the Palero can communicate with; Iroko's roots are the home of a powerful spirit called *Mama Ungungu*. Soil from around Iroko is offered to the orishas *Oddua and Brazo Fuerte*. A tea made from Iroko's leaves will open a neophyte's third eye and help her become a spirit medium. The spirit of Iroko can be contacted even if the tree is not present by singing the mambo listed above while shaking an iroko stick rythmically in front of the nganga.

THE EVIL EYE

A small piece of Iroko wood hung with a red ribbon by a baby's crib will protect her from the evil eye. Since we Paleros believe that there is an eternal struggle between the forces of good and the forces of evil, we have a responsibility to learn how to combat evil in order to maximize our happiness and that of our loved ones.

The evil eye is a natural manifestation of evil. Knowing that the eyes are the windows of the soul, we can surmise that a perverted, sick individual who has allowed his soul to become tainted with evil will sometimes even unwittingly look at someone and this evil will spill from his soul through his eyes, affecting the person he is looking at in a negative fashion. Because of their innocence, babies are particularly vulnerable to the evil eye and must be protected at all times. Because they are most defenseless while they sleep, babies should not be allowed to be looked upon while they are asleep. If a stranger or a person known for his evil eye compliments your baby, make sure he utters the phrase *"may God bless her"* right after. Otherwise, you must say to yourself the words *"besale el culito, besale el culito, besale el culito . . ."* several times. This literally means *"kiss his little ass,"* why it works, no one knows.

Other talismans against the evil eye that work are a piece of jet *(azabache)*, a piece of red coral, or a dog's tooth. Although many Hispanic jewellers in the U.S. claim they sell azabaches, many times they are selling black plastic beads instead. Genuine jet does not shine, can be pierced with a needle, and will stain a white paper black if one runs it across it. Other implements successfully used to ward off the evil eye are garlic, camphor, and a prayer to St. Louis Bertand (San Luis Beltran). The great Palero Andres Petit, founder of the Kimbisa faction of Palo, said there was no more powerful defense against the evil eye than the prayer to San Luis Beltran. He always carried it with him and would write it down for any one who asked—he knew it by heart.

PRAYER OF SAINT LUIS BELTRAN

*Creature of God, I exorcize, treat, and bless you
in the name of the Holy Trinity.*

Father , Son , and Holy Spirit , Three different persons and one true essence; and of the Virgin Mary, Our Lady, conceived without stain of original sin. Virgin before giving birth , during birth V, and after the birth V, by the glorious St. Gertrude, your beloved and given spouse, by the Eleven Thousand Virgins, by Saint Joseph, Saint Rocco, and Saint Sebastian, and by all the saints of your celestial court, by your Very Glorious Incarnation, Very Glorious Birth, Very Holy Passion, Very Glorious Resurrection, and Divine Ascencion. By so high and holy mysteries that I in truth believe, I plead to your Divine Majesty, placing as intercessessor your Divine Mother, Our Advocate, that you liberate and heal this afflicted creature of any sickness, evil eye, pain, accident, or fever, or any any other injury, wound, or malady, Amen Jesus.

Not looking at the unworthy person who would prefer such sacrosanct mysteries, with such good faith I plead to you, oh Lord, for your greater glory and devotion of those present, that you will by your piety and mercy heal or liberate from this wound, affliction, pain, humor, sickness, taking it away from this part and place. And may your Divine Majesty not allow accident, corruption, or injury to overcome him, giving him health so that, with it, he may serve you and fulfill your Most Holy Will. Amen Jesus.

I exorcize and treat you, and Jesus Christ Our Lord heals you, blesses you, and lets unfold his Divine Will. Amen Jesus.

Consumatum est, Consumatum est , Consumatum est .

LOWERING A FEVER

Andres also gave my father the following *recipe for lowering a fever:* Arrange for three people to read the prayer to San Luis by the bed of the feverish person. Each reader must come, read the prayer, and leave without seeing who read before or after, and all three must read in turn not more than one hour apart. A little cross made out of basil leaves and holy water from a Catholic church must also be used by the reader, who must sprinkle some holy water on the feverish person while making the sign of the cross over the him or her while holding the basil cross pressed between the right index finger and the thumb each time it says to do so in the written prayer.

A SPECIAL BAPTISMAL WATER

A special chamba made out of the leaves of Iroko, guara, yaya, tengue, and caja, serves as baptismal water for infants. Babies baptized in this chamba, called Mamba Nsanbi, grow strong and healthy. Let it be clear that infant baptism in Palo does not make our children Paleros. They will choose if they wish to remain in Palo when they are old enough to make such a decision.

CHAPTER 4

THE MAKING OF A NGANGA

Nganga means "mystery," "soul," or "force." In Africa, what we call a Palo priest is called a "Nganga." In Cuba, nganga refers to the cauldron which is at the center of our practice. This cauldron is also called *"prenda,"* which in Old Spanish meant "precious," implying that the nganga is dear to us. The making of a nganga involves the signing of a pact between a living being and one who has passed on to the spirit world. A spirit who agrees to work with a Palero in this fashion is called a *"nganga luzambi"* or *"nganga ndoki."* The making of a nganga involves going to the bush and to the cemetery, contracting with a spirit, and knowing how to control that spirit.

In the cemetery one finds the human remains needed for the nganga; in the bush the plants and spirits one needs to contact. Cemetery and bush are not that different, in both one finds the *Nfumbi,* souls willing to make a pact with the Palero. A nganga may be inherited, but more often it is specially made by the padrino for the new ngangulero. In old munanzos, it would take at least seven years after "scratching" for a Palero to be considered for ngangulero. Because of the exigencies of modern life, the time has been shortened to one year and seven days in most munanzos.

The Padrino *"monta"* (makes) the nganga by putting inside the cauldron the bones, vines, sticks, herbs, soils, animal carcasses, and other secret ingredients which give the nganga life. Every nganga must have an *otan* (stone) or *piedra de rayo* (stone arrowhead), also called *matari*. These dark, flat, elongated stones are pointed on one end and have white streaks running through them. They are sacred to Siete Rayos. Siete Rayos, by the way, is a corruption of Cetewayo, the famous Zulu chief, nephew of Shaka, thought to be an incarnation of the god of thunder. The stone must be fed sacrificial blood, *menga,* separately. Then it "eats" again when the entire nganga is fed. Ceremonies of initiation should be done either during the new moon, *tangu or oshuka guamiaku,* or during the full moon, *oshuka dida.* Never during waning moon, *oshuka aro,* a time when plants lose their powers. The following prayer is offered to the new moon:

> *Luna nueva, yo te saludo, dame salud, tranquilidad al mundo, que no haya guerra, ni enfermedad, aqui te doy una moneda pa'que no nos falte el pan ni a mi ni a mis hijos, familiares, amigos, y enemigos.*

Afterwards three "Our Fathers," three "Ave Marias," and one "Gloria" are recited, followed by the following Lukumi prayer:

> *Chukwa madeni*
> *Ochukwa made rawo*
> *Ochukwa madeni*
> *Ochukwa made rawo*
> *Solodde guini guini eco eco*
> *Ochukwa imabere inawo*
> *Inawo ima were*

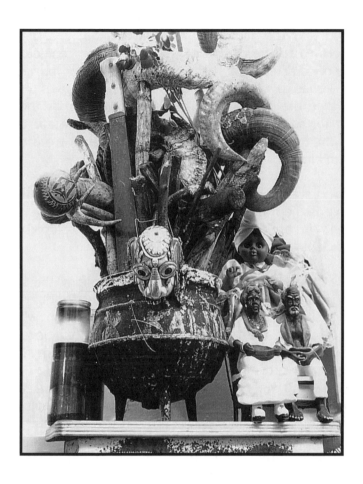

(Fig.3) The terrifying nganga Camposanto Medianoche, bursting with animal skulls, rams' horns, machetes and sticks. Note the statues of an old man and woman, representing the archetypal ancestral African Spirits "Francisco and Francisca."

Mother Moon is godmother to all magicians. She is the queen of all heavenly bodies. The Moon presides over a ngangulero's initiation. She is *"Mama Mposi,"* the *"All-Mother."* It is during the full moon that the godfather, the *mayordomo,* and the future ngangulero go to the cemetery, asking with the chomolongos or with the obi oracle at the foot of each grave if that *muerto* (dead person) wishes to work with them. If the oracle gives a positive answer, then the padrino spills some rum *(malafo)* by the grave, listening for some rumbling sounds which will indicate that the spirit of the dead body buried under the chosen grave is eager to work with him.

The next step is to form a cross over the grave using the rum. The grave is then dug up and the *kiyumba* (skull), fingers, toes, tibias, and ribs are removed from the cadaver and placed inside a large black bag.

Back at the munanzo, the black bag containing the bones is covered with a white sheet as four white candles are lit around it. The padrino then calls out the name of the dead person, which had been copied from the tombstone at the gravesite. Seven small piles of gunpowder *(fula)* are placed on top of one of the flat sides of a large sugar-cutting knife called a machete. If they all explode at the same time when fire is applied to one of them, it means that the spirit (nfumbi) has agreed to become the resident spirit of the nganga that is being made.

Using a pencil, the padrino then writes the name of the nfumbi on a piece of parchment or brown paper bag, placing it at the bottom of the cauldron that will become the new ngangulero's prenda. The padrino now adds to the name the dead man's bones, seven silver coins, the previously prepared stone, and a razor blade (preferably the one that had been used to cut scratches on the new ngangulero's skin). A black chicken or rooster is now offered to the nganga-in-the-making to ensure the continuing well-being of the proceedings. Other sacrifices also take place at this time.

Further ingredients that go into the nganga are: *soil taken from four different spots surrounding the grave*(North, South, East, and West), *a hollowed piece of bamboo* about two inches in diameter and six to twelve inches long that had been previously filled with mercury, sea water, and sand from a beach, all of which had been sealed inside with beeswax; *the remains of a small black male dog* which will serve as the nfumbi's pet and messenger, *dirt from an anthill, the necessary twenty-one foundation sticks* (sold as a package in most major botanicas in the U.S.), *termites, a dead bat, spiders, lizards, a centipede, a toad, cinnamon, chili peppers, ginger, a white onion, sage, and more soil from the grave.* The cauldron is then taken to the cemetery, where it is buried on a Friday in a spot where it won't be disturbed, preferably close to the grave of the nfumbi. The nganga is left buried for three weeks.

After three weeks have elapsed, the nganga is dug up, a chicken is sacrificed on the spot and nine pennies are left on the hole left by the removal of the nganga. This is a symbolic payment to the forces that govern the cemetery and a reminder that one doesn't receive anything in this world without paying for it. The nganga is immediately taken to the bush, where it is buried next to Iroko or another sacred tree and left there for another three weeks.

After three more weeks have passed, the cauldron is removed from that spot and, after the spirit of the tree has been offered a chicken and eight pennies (or six if it is a palm tree), the cauldron is taken to the munanzo. It is placed next to the temple's main nganga and left there for three more weeks in order for it to receive ashé (strength). At the end of these three weeks, a black rooster whose throat is slit but is not decapitated is offered as a sacrifice. *Rum, nutmeg, dry white wine, and Florida Water* are then added to the nganga, that is now ready to occupy its place of honor in the new ngangulero's home.

A traditional type of nganga not usually made anymore is the *nganga boumba*, which uses a burlap bag as its receptacle, rather than a cauldron. This nganga requires as ingredients the twenty-one foundation sticks, the legs, heads, and hearts from the following animals: a dog, a cat, an opossum (a rat can be substituted), a black goat, a sparrow, an owl, a bat, a vulture, a woodpecker, a blackbird, and a parrot. Plus the remains of a snake, a lizard, a toad, a frog, a tarantula a scorpion, a centipede, a wasp, a dragonfly, red ants, termites, worms, and caterpillars. Originally, all evil prendas were kept in burlap bags, not in cauldrons since the cauldron, as a representative of the justice-loving god Zarabanda, does not lend itself well to undeserved evil. The boumba, also called *sacu-sacu*, was kept hanging by a rope from the padrino's ceiling. The padrino had to sing the following mambo to the sacu-sacu before lowering it to the floor:

> *Ay Lembe Lembe Lembe*
> *Mi caballo 'ta 'tropiao*
> *Malembe yaya*
> *Lembe Lembe Malembe*
> *Andale siete legua*
> *Que yo vengo*
> *Cuando llegue aqui*
> *Lembe Lembe Malembe*
> *Siete legua que yo vengo*
> *Gurubana con licensia*
> *Jacinto congo ta la loma*

These burlap ngangas were also called *"macutos."* Before bringing down the sacu-sacu, the padrino would also sweep the floor under it with much ceremony while singing the following mambo:

> *Barre, barre, barre, basura*
> *Barre, barre, barre, basura*
> *Simbico, Simbico*
> *Tata Nganga ya limpio piso*

The Tata would then sign his firma (sygill) on the floor using ashes or white chalk *(cascarrilla or pembe).* The Tata would also draw the traditional Palo sign for the universe *(see below),* afterwards singing the following mambo:

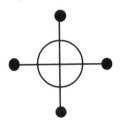

Mpati! Mpati!
Npembe Simbi ko?
Mpati! Mpati!
Npembe Simbi ko, Simbi ko?
Como Tata te mando
Abajo nganga
Bajalo, mi Mama
Como Tata te mando
Bajalo, mi Mama
Trailo, trailo, mi nganga
Trailo, nganga, como paso l'inguana
Despacio como anda camaleon

The sticks were then carefully taken out of the bag and placed leaning by a wall in a vertical, standing position. While this operation was undertaken, the Tata would sing the following mambo.

Paralo, paralo mi Mama
Como Tata te mando
Paralo, paralo, Simbico
Pa'que yo jura mi Mama
Simbico, paralo.

While continuing to organize the contents of the sacu-sacu, the padrino would continue singing:

> *Yaya patempolo*
> *pa'to lo mundo Simbico*
> *Yaya patempolo*
> *Yaya Maria Nganga*
> *Ya vamo a ve' Simbico*
> *Que patimpolo goya ya que patimpolo*
> *Mambe Dios*
> *Mambe Dios*

Once the sacu-sacu was organized on the floor, the Tata and his assistant would proceed to spray rum or aguardiente on it, also offering the nganga cigar smoke while singing:

> *Sala mi nganga, sala la o*
> *Nsunga de vuelta ligenia*
> *Arriba mundo to mocua*
> *Singa, vamo'nsunga*
> *Yimbila, yimbila*

Immediately afterwards, the Tata would sing the following:

> *Mayombe fue bueno en guinea*
> *Con lonyaya, lonyaya*
> *Cuando viene,*
> *Vamo a ve*
> *Susundama ya ta pinta nganga*
> *Mayombe bueno en Guinea*
> *Mama Lola da licensia*
> *Abre camino*
> *Mayombe fue bueno en Guinea*
> *Mayombe abre camino*
> *Chikirungoma recogi*
> *Chikirungoma a recoge*
> *Vamo recoge*

After working with the sacu-sacu, the Tata would carefully place everything back inside the burlap bag and hang the nganga back from the ceiling. Such was the way of the sacu-sacu nganga in the days of old.

The life of each nganga is sustained by the sticks (palos) of the bush *(nfinda)* that give our religion its name, by the spirit who has chosen to reside in it, and by all of the animals it contains. A nganga is a micro-universe reflecting all that one can find in the larger world, both good and evil. This is why so many ingredients go into a nganga, because it must reflect the forces of the universe, forces that are channeled in a nganga to be used by the ngangulero, who is like the god of the nganga. Since Andres Petit initiated whites into Palo back in the mid 1840s, members of virtually all races and nationalities have discovered this path which, while it is not for everyone, everyone can benefit from it.

A strong mind is needed to guide a nganga well. I believe the spirits of former slaves that usually work with nganguleros like to test us. They also have a tendency to try to obtain revenge from whites because of the mistreatment they may have received while in their last incarnation. Nganguleros have a responsibility not to give in to these feelings of revenge, instead channeling that energy towards less destructive aims. I believe good is good and bad is bad. No one race has a monopoly on either, so lets move on.

There is only one way to destroy a nganga. After feeding it the blood of a rooster, rum, and cigar smoke, bury it beneath an anthill saying loudly "GOOD BYE FOREVER!" If, however, other ngangas have been born from that one, the parent nganga will continue to exist in an ethereal form as long as its descendants exist. To be a ngangulero, a person must have a stable character, a strong mind, faith in God and the orishas, respect and obedience for his padrino, and the humility to realize that to be placed in a position of leadership in the world of spirits is a huge responsibility as well as a great privilege.

CHAPTER 5

Nkisis, Kimpungulu: The Deities

NGURUFINDA / BURUFINDA / OSAIN

We start with Ngurufinda(Burufinda), also known in Palo as Sindaula Ndundu and Yembaka Butanseke, called Osain in Lukumi, because as god of plants he is vary close to every Palero's heart. It is said that Osain began the practice of making magical potions out of plants and storing the potions in gourds and calabashes many, many, years ago. It was a woman who first discovered the secret potions, forcing Burufinda to share knowledge of how to work with herbs with the woman. She in turn promised not to work with herbs while on her menses, which rendered her ritualistically unclean, a promise she did not keep. Since that time, most Paleros have taboos against giving the Burufinda deity to women. In our house, we make special osains for women called Osain Kinibos, these are kept outside the home and must be hung at a low altitude, less than eight feet.

People born with the gift of working with plants are called "Osainistas" and are usually children of Siete Rayos (Shangó), Osain's favorite godchild. It was to Shangó that Osain first taught the secret of how to make powerful medicine out of plants and it was he who first kept a gourd filled with a magical potion in his home. Lucero, Zarabanda, Vence Batallas, and the nfumbi are all intimately intertwined with Burufinda/Osain. The Osain we work with in our house is called Osain Aguenegui Agualdo Kinikini and the way to praise him is with the following mambo:

> *Oile sai sai babalogwo*
> *Oile sai sai babalogwo*
> *Osain aweneye eli se ko*
> *Ewel'eye n'ile 'yare obaniwe*

Osain eats goats, tortoises, and roosters, especially fighting roosters and those called *"silky."* Ingredients for a gourd Osain include deer antlers, soil from at least seven different places, sticks, a tortoise that has been sacrificed to Osain, rain water collected in May, sea water, river water, Catholic holy water, and whole pepper kernels which must be chewed and spat inside the gourd by the tata. The Osain deity also requires bugs, birds, and coins. After the gourd is filled with all these ingredients, it is then taken to a palm tree, where it is buried for six days in order to receive Siete Rayos' and his sister Dada's ashé. By burying Osain for eight days next to Iroko, Tiembla-Tierra, Nana Bukuu, and Aganju imbues it with power. Kept buried for three days in an anthill gives the Osain deity the blessings of the nfumbis, while burying it for three days in a crossroads gives it power from Lucero. Each time Osain is taken out of the earth (tilé) a rooster, a tortoise, toasted corn, dry wine, a silver coin, and rum, must be left inside the hole, and a Catholic prayer called *"The Apostles Creed"* as well as the *"Our Father"* must be recited after each removal of Osain from a burial. This is called "thanking the earth." Some Osains are not made in gourds, but in terra cotta dishes or small iron cauldrons.

The secret powder that gives life to Osain can be kept inside a small bottle, inside an antler, inside a bull or cow horn, or inside a little gourd. Divination determines which will be used. This powder is made out of four feet from a tortoise, two feet from a small parrot, the remains of a large parrot or macaw, the remains of a turtle dove, the following sticks: amansa-guapo, wakibanza, sapo; plus the eyes and tongue of a rooster, seven large ants, seven human teeth which include the two canines, dirt from a graveyard, hair from a dead person, the name of the same dead person written on parchment, seven mate seeds, plus a little rum. All of these ingredients are to be burned to a crisp, the ashes that remain, along with some stuff that didn't burn, is put on a mortar and ground with a pestle to a powder. The ensuing powder is a powerful ashé that is stored in one of the receptacles described above and then placed inside the larger gourd that had been prepared before. On a Thursday, Friday, or Saturday, the whole deity is to be buried along with a large piece of Iroko, sacrificing another turtle at the site. Three weeks later the Osain is ready to be taken out. The Osain is now complete, ready to be hung up high from the ceiling or from a tree in your backyard or patio, a practice I don't recommend because your enemies may have access to this precious nkisi if it is outside.

LUCERO MUNDO / TATA NKUYU / ESHU / ELEGGUA

Also called *Tata Nfinda and Quicio-Puerta*. Lucero is THE CHILD, a natural trickster. He is easily irritable and must be cared for. Like any child, Lucero does not respond well to neglect. He is the most indispensable of the orishas, for without him nothing moves. He is called *el portero*, the gatekeeper, for without his blessing no metaphysical doorway can be entered, and, without his help, no material threshold can be crossed. With his cowry shells, a priest can address any orisha. It is his shells that serve best for in-depth readings. Lucero enjoys offerings of toys, candy, and all those things dear to children. He enjoys parties and celebrations, as well as games. Lucero is a happy-go-lucky youth, yet he can be brutal if one forgets to propitiate him on Mondays. Lucero may forgive the Palero if he forgets to honor him once or twice, but if a third week goes by without Lucero receiving his tribute, then the Palero will be reminded that he needs Lucero by losing a lot of business.

To honor Lucero on Mondays, offer him rum sprayed on the Lucero figure directly from your mouth, cigar smoke, a candle, and a clear glass of water. Remember to talk to Lucero throughout your Monday ceremony, telling him step-by-step what you are doing: *"I am now lighting a candle for you, my precious child, I will now spray some rum on you, beloved Lucero,"* etc. Speak to him sweetly, as if you were speaking to a child. Always remind him that he is the lord of your home. Before addressing him, always knock three times on the floor in front of Lucero, using the knuckles of your right hand.

Lucero is one of the Warriors and is often kept next to Zarabanda, Oshosi and Osun. Osun, not to be confused with Oshun, is a nkisi associated with Osain, representing the Practitioner as a deity, a reminder of the inherent godhood within us all. Osun is depicted as a little metal rooster standing in what looks like a chalice. In Africa, Osun is a metal staff as tall as the practitioner, capped by a bird, and stuck in the ground in front of a practitioner's home. This tells people that a Tata lives on the premises.

MAKING LUCERO

*(**Warning:** Only duly initiated tatas, santeros, orisha priests, babalawos, houngans, or other priesthood holders at a similar level have the necessary ashé to make an efficacious Lucero deity—it is dangerous for the non-initiated to attempt to make a Lucero. What the un-initiated can do in order to have a temporary Lucero is take a coconut, dress it with palm oil, and place it behind his/her door, honoring it as a Lucero.)*

To make a Lucero deity, a stone the size and approximate shape of a potato is chosen by divination. The stone is bathed in chamba.

At the bottom of the stone, with cement mixed with chamba, stick several nickels that have been obtained from different, successful, businesses such as banks. Add copper coins, a piece of silver, a piece of gold, dust from inside and outside the main door of the person who is to receive the Lucero, soil from outside a grocery store, dirt from a crossroads, and other ingredients such as mercury and pieces of kola nuts. Eyes, nose, and mouth fashioned out of cowry shells can be glued on to the stone. A chicken is then sacrificed allowing its blood (menga) to flow over the deity while songs to Lucero are sung. Afterwards Lucero is buried in a crossroads for a total of twenty-one days, after he is unearthed, the hole that remains must be filled with a sacrifice.

Lucero is then brought to the house in which he'll stay, a party having been organized in his honor. Lucero loves palm oil, honey, dry white wine, dried fish, dried possum, candy, rum, cigar smoke, cool water, and a candle.

Before a person receives a Lucero from a padrino or madrina, both parties should be aware that this exchange makes them responsible to each other, since after a padrino confers a Lucero on someone, that person is forever to be considered the padrino's godchild. People who do not respect each other or do not get along should not enter into a godparent/godchild relationship, for there is a Kikongo proverb that says *"it is better to be torn apart by four elephants and eaten by ten vultures and seventeen hyenas than to speak badly of one's godfather."* A godchild's disrespect for a godparent will be punished by the orishas, but a godparent's abuse of his or her godchild will also receive punishment.

The following are Lucero's attributes:

Colors: Red and black
Fruits: Guava, sugar cane
Herb: Pasture
Beverages: Aguardiente, rum, dry white wine
Mineral: Jet

Animals: Chicken, small goats, rooster, chick
Condiment: Palm oil
Stick: Abre-camino
Numbers: 3, 21

Lucero is lord of the lonely death; he kills those who deserve it by making them bleed to death. Lucero loves parties, food, and sweets. When entering a place where a Lucero deity is present, the initiate will salute Lucero with the following praise:

*Eshu a ke buru bori ake boye to ri to ru la
ye fi yo'ru a're a la le ku'pa she eyo me'ko*

Lucero should be petitioned to keep away evil in the following manner:

Ko si iku	*keep away death*
Ko si ofo	*keep away loss*
Ko si araye	*keep away tragedy*
Ko si ewan	*keep away prison*
Ko si fitibo	*keep away obstacles*
Ko si ashelu	*keep away the police*
Ko si egba	*keep away paralysis*
Ko si arun	*keep away illness*

Lucero is humankind's teacher par excellence, always putting people through tests. Lucero has twenty-one manifestations in Palo, but all are one. The oldest Lucero is called Elufe. He is fashioned out of wood and goes inside the Nganga. Elufe has 21 "sons" or "caminos "(paths); these are:

1. Kunanmembe, "He who is just as well good as bad."
2. Prima, "Lucero at dawn or dusk."
3. Ndaya, "Lord of the Netherworld."
4. Pitilanga, "Lord of the Seashore."
5. Madruga, "Lord of the wee hours of morning."
6. Aprueba-fuerza, "Lord of the Rails."

7. Vence Guerra, "Winner of Battles."
8. Vira-Mundo, "World-turner."
9. Monteoscuro, "Lord of Dark Mountains."
10. Busca Buya lives at the police station.
11. Mundo Nuevo protects prisoners.
12. Rompe Monte, the Lucero that is represented by a terra-cotta roof tile.
13. Sabicunanguasa, the Lucero who lives at the river's banks and eats black hens.
14. Talatarde, Lord of Pestilence.
15. Katilemba, Kubayende's sidekick.
16. Casco Duro, Lucero of the Lakes.
17. Tronco Malva, Lord of the Four Cardinal Points.
18. Pata Sueno, "Lord of the Crossroads."
19. Jaguey Grande, Lord of the Mountains.
20. Kabankiriyo, Lord of Darkness. ,
21. Siete Puertas, Lord of the Underdog.

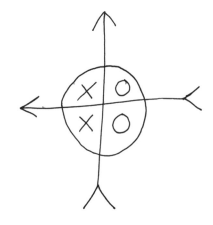

1. Lucero Kunanmembe:

The most versatile sygill. May be used for any purpose.

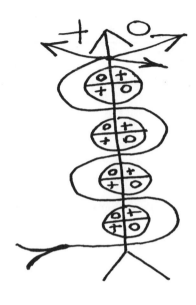

2. Lucero Prima:
Paint this sygill outside a bottle and keep an evil soul trapped there.

3. Lucero Ndaya:
Draw this sygill with white or yellow chalk to protect a dwelling.

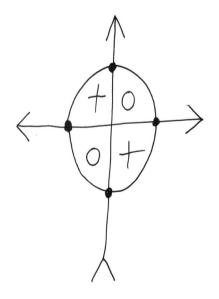

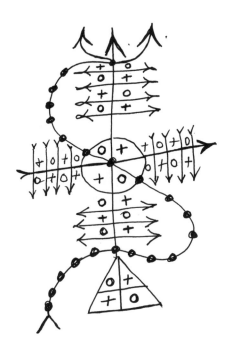

4. Lucero Pitilanga:

The following verse was written in English by Andres Petit himself.

"On Good Friday at nightfall draw this sign and call evil to obey you. Now and then feed the sign an old black hen."

5. Lucero Madrugá:

An effective sygill when invoking the spirits of dead tatas.

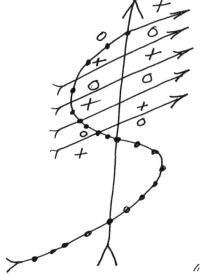

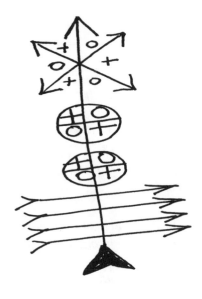

6. Lucero Aprueba Fuerza:

Draw this sygill before invoking Zarabanda.

7. Lucero Vence Batalla:

Draw this sygill to win any battle.

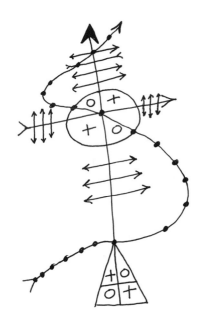

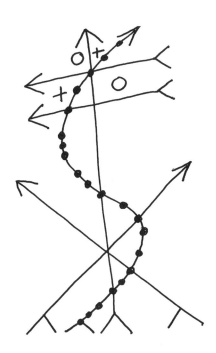

8. Lucero Vira Mundo:
Draw this sygill to
break any spell.

9. Lucero Monte Oscuro:
Draw this sygill when ready to
engage in a dangerous battle.

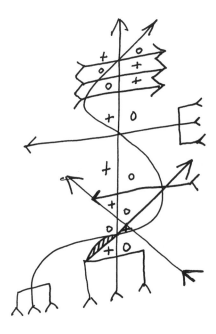

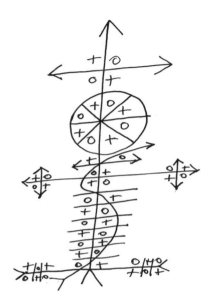

10. Lucero Busca Buya:
Keeps the police away.

11. Lucero Mundo Nuevo:
Use to get someone out
of prison.

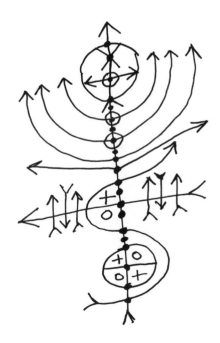

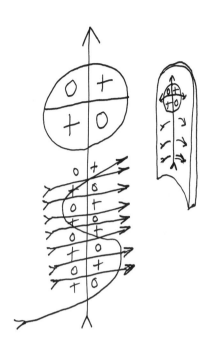

12. Lucero Rompe Monte:
Feed it a snake and ask that it turns someone crazy.

13. Lucero Sabi Kunanguasa:
Kill him a black hen at the bank of a river and he will grant you a wish.

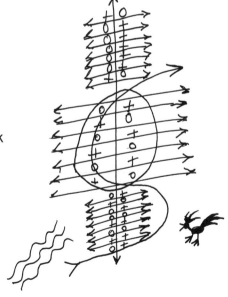

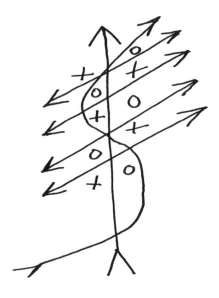

14. Lucero Tala Tarde:
Place nine different types of herbs in a bottle of Chamba, draw this sygill next to your Nganga and refresh it with the chamba.

15. Lucero Katilemba:
Kubayende's sidekick.

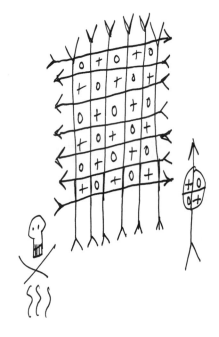

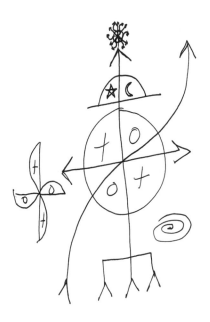

16.Lucero Casco Duro:
Sacrifice a chicken to this
sygill by a lake for health
and good fortune.

17. Lucero Tronco Malva:
" To protect and defend", is this
lucero's maxim.

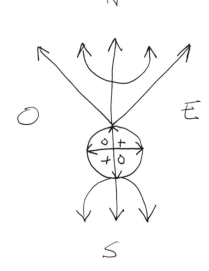

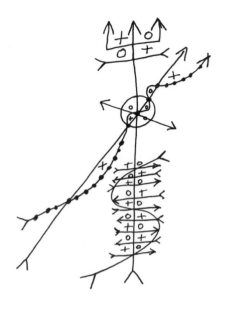

18. Lucero Patasueño:
Draw this sygill before embarking on a trip to ensure success.

19. Lucero Jaguey Grande:
Draw this sygill when you want to invoke the spirits of the forest.

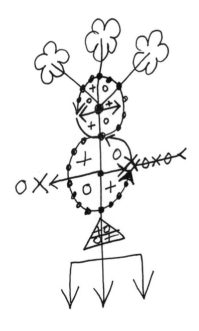

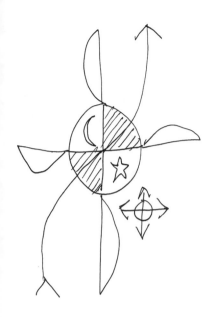

20. Lucero Kabankiriyo:
Use this sygill to attack enemies.

21. Lucero Siete Puertas:
Works with the Dead. Lives at the gates of the cemetery.

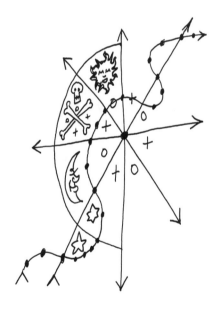

TIEMBLA-TIERRA / KENGUE / OBATALÁ

Owner of everything white, protector of albinos, said to be his legitimate children. Creator of human heads (intelligence). Tiembla-Tierra brought fertility to the world by splitting into male and female halves, thus introducing sexual intercourse into the world. Most orishas were born to this primordial couple.

The following are Tiembla-Tierra's attributes:

Color: White
Fruits: Soursop, cantaloupe
Herb: jasmine
Beverages: water, milk
Mineral: Platinum, white marble
Animals: White doves, white she-goats
Condiment: Cocoa butter
Stick: Silk-cotton
Numbers: 8, 24

SIETE RAYOS / NSASI / SHANGÓ

Arguably the most popular of all Palo deities, my father told me that this deity was actually a real king in South Africa named Cetewayo who lived in the late 1800s and was considered an incarnation of the god of thunder. Siete Rayos does not like the dead, for his vibrant personality loves everything sensual such as drumming, dancing, fighting and copulating. He lives on the top of the extremely tall royal palm trees.

The following are Siete Rayo's attributes:

Colors: Red and white
Fruits: Red bananas, red apples
Herb: Palm frond
Beverages: Aguardiente, rum, red wine

Mineral: Stone arrowheads; ruby
Animals: Rooster, goat, quail
Condiment: Palm oil
Stick: palm
 Numbers: 4, 6

Men must not mistreat daughters of Siete Rayos, for the god fiercely protects his female devotees. The following mambo is sung to Siete Rayos:

Abukenke jugo con lo'Sambi
Yo no va casa lo'santo
Zarabanda son mi zapato
Lucero son mi camisa
y a el si lo acato enseguida
Siete Rayos son bendito

All Paleros worship Siete Rayos, even those dedicated to evil. He is considered the first Palero, the greatest magician, the king of our religion. Another mambo to Siete Rayos goes like this:

Matari Nsasi, matari mukiana
Matari monovelo es la envoltura
La piedra en que Nkita Nsasi cae del cielo
Nsasi mura nsulu
Fula inoka muinda
Muna nsulu sucrila
Nsasi kimfunla inumantato
Nsasi 'ta en cielo
Estrella, cae en tierra, y baja.

This mambo talks about how Siete Rayos rules the heavens, sending lightning to his enemies, lording over all heavenly bodies. Siete Rayos is the most attractive of all male Nkisis.

MADRE DE AGUA / MAMA KALUNGA / YEMAYÁ

First-born of Tiembla-Tierra, wife of Brazo Fuerte, Mother of Humanity. Madre de Agua rules the oceans from where all life emerged. She is said to possess wisdom as vast as the ocean, and can offer her devotees unimaginable riches.

The following are Madre de Agua's attributes:

> **Colors:** Blue and white (her necklace consist of blue and clear beads)
> **Fruit:** Watermelon
> **Herb:** Seaweed
> **Beverages:** Aguardiente, molasses
> **Mineral:** Aquamarine
> **Animals:** Ducks, roosters, sheep
> **Condiment:** Molasses
> **Stick:** Bamboo
> **Numbers:** 7, 12

MAMA SHOLA WANGUE / MPUNGU / OSHÚN

Orisha of beauty, very vibrant, known for her expansive laughter. She is the goddess of love, but is also a fierce warrior. Mama Shola rules all rivers. She loves her devotees, but can be brutal with them if they fail to meet her expectations. Once Mama Shola turns against a devotee, she may never forgive him. Mama Shola demands that promises made to her be kept. Priests who work with Mama Shola must be paid in advance and in full for their services.

The following are Mama Shola Wangue's attributes:

> **Colors:** Yellow and amber
> **Fruits:** Oranges, yellow cantaloupes
> **Herb:** Chamomile
> **Beverage:** Beer

Mineral: Gold, copper, amber (not really a mineral,
but functioning as one)
Animals: Castrated goats, yellow hens
Condiment: Honey
Stick: Cinnamon
Number: 5

ZARABANDA / CHIBIRIKI / OGÚN

Owner of iron, so respected in those parts of Africa that worship him that to swear on him is accepted in court as equivalent to swearing on the Bible or the Holy Qur'an. He is one of four nkisis collectively called "The Warriors." Zarabanda is present where ever iron is found, he is therefore almost always found in ngangas, since most are contained in iron cauldrons. To prepare a Zarabanda deity, the following ingredients must be gathered: A stone picked out in the wilderness, certain human bones, soil, a horseshoe, handcuffs, an iron chain, an iron ball, mercury, two bottles of rum, dry white wine, cigars, and a pigeon. A small black dog must be sacrificed, his skull being kept forever in the cauldron. The ritual of making Zarabanda must begin at midnight. The vulture, mayimbe, must be praised by singing, "Dió, Dió, Dió Mayimbe, Mayimbe, Mayimbe."

When you go forth to the wilderness in order to find the required stone needed for Zarabanda, take an egg as an offering. When you see a blackish or gray stone that catches your eye, take it. The following sticks are indispensable to Zarabanda: palo hueso, palo jiqui, quiebra hacha, malambo and palo yaya. Another feature that must not be overlooked In Zarabanda's prenda is the addition of a heavy, padlocked chain which is wound tightly around the outer rim of the cauldron and is said to function as a barrier to keep Zarabanda's enormous energy inside the cauldron until the Palero is ready to use it. Zarabanda's firma (see bellow) is painted outside and inside the cauldron. The cauldron is then covered with a black and white cloth after a possum, jutia, or guinea pig,

65

plus a black rooster, has been sacrificed to Zarabanda. It is then buried near Iroko or another sacred tree for twenty-one days, feeding the earth appropriately after the cauldron has been unearthed. This is the mambo that has to be sung while making Zarabanda:

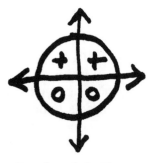

Zarabanda's Firma

Yo mimo cheche
Que kuenda ntoto
Tu kuenda la finda
Tu kuenda carabasa
Ndoki que yo bobba
Tu mimo son mi pare
Tu mimo son mi mare
Tu mimo son to lankan
Mo Ko jumansen kiyumba

The cauldron is now ready. Zarabanda's firma is now drawn on the floor or table where the deity will be placed. The circle represents the world, each point of the cross represents a cardinal point, and the center of the cross represents the crossroads—choices. Seven piles of gunpowder are lit to welcome Zarabanda to its home, the new owner of the nganga may now decorate it with vulture feathers. A cat bone—usually the tailbone—is sometimes added to Zarabanda. Pick the right bone by placing a magic mirror near it, if it gets cloudy, that is the bone you'll choose.

The following are Zarabanda's attributes:

Colors: Green and black; white and black in some
munanzos, red in others
Fruit or tuber: African yam, green plantain
Herb: Ginger, lemongrass
Beverage: Zarabanda loves hard liquor, but should
only be offered some on special occasions
Mineral: Iron

Animals: Dogs, young bulls
Condiment: Black pepper
Stick: Algarrobo
Number: 3, 7

PATA-EN-LLAGA / KUBAYENDE / BABALÚ AIYE

A terrifying entity in Africa, where he is known as the one who brings plagues, in the Americas he has been truly syncretized with the beloved old beggar depicted in Catholic lithographs accompanied by two small dogs that lick the sores which cover his body. Pata-en-llaga was born lame, showing us that even the gods may be faced with physical challenges. In fact, Pata-en-llaga had to overcome not one, but several disabilities, including severe skin problems, syphillis, and ignorance of the language and customs of the land to where he was sent as an exile, Arará. Because of his indomitable spirit and his enormous strength of character, Babalú has become the most beloved orisha in Cuba, the people of our country identifying with this great fighter who went from royal prince to exiled criminal to king of his own land. Pata-en-llaga's perseverance becomes emblematic of the Cuban ethos. Syncretized with St. Lazarus, not the friend of Jesus, but the old man of the parable of the rich man and the poor man, on December 17th massive pilgrimages to a little church outside Havana which houses a miraculous image of the alleged saint (theologians will tell you that parables are allegories, so this particular Lazarus probably never existed). People from all parts of Cuba and from all walks of life and religious traditions walk, crawl, or ride to the little church and leprosarium where Pata-en-llaga/Babalú is said to reside disguised as an old white man on crutches.

The following are Pata-en-llaga's attributes:

Colors: Purple, brown, yellow
Fruits: Dates, raisins
Herb: Escoba amarga, apazote
Beverage: Dry white wine; milk for his dogs
Mineral: Quartz
Animals: Guinea fowl, castrated goats
Condiment: Sesame seeds
Stick: Arbol del sebo
Number: 11, 13, 17

Pata-en-llaga protects the elderly, people with skin conditions, people with blood infections, graveyard workers, pimps, dogs, and the poor. Burlap is another one of his attributes, it reminds Pata-en-llaga of a time when he was so poor he had to dress himself by fashioning clothes out of discarded burlap bags. A common sacrifice offered to Pata-en-llaga after he grants a boon is for the devotee to dress in burlap, either for a prolonged period, such as a month, or for one day per month, usually on the 17th.

A simple way to honor Pata-en-llaga is to take a toasted or dried corn-on-the cob, such as the kind sold in the U.S. as ornamentation during Halloween, dress it with palm oil, attach seven different-colored ribbons, each about a foot in length, from the cob, and hang it inside your home from the middle of your front door. Nail a piece of bread or dinner roll right above the corn-on-the cob so that you'll never lack food and prosperity.

CENTELLA NDOKI / MARIWANGA / OYA

The fiercest female warrior and beloved wife of Siete Rayos, Centella Ndoki rules over Nfuiri, the Angel of Death--known as Ikú in Santeria. Centella Ndoki protects merchants, as she is called *"La Dueña de la Plaza"*(The owner of the marketplace). She is said to be present at the gates of cemeteries. This indicates that part of her role is to aid people who are making the transition from the material to the spiritual plane. Along with her sisters Mama Shola Wanga and Mama Kalunga, she rules over waters, her particular dominion being rainwater. Her power as a mediator is also evident here, for she not only rules over rainwater, but also over lightning, which is fire. Centella Ndoki's most important aspect, however, is as the ruler of the wind, especially storms. Her dominion of air implies that she is one of the forces that sustains life, for there can be no life as we know it without the air we breath. All of these attributes make Centella Ndoki, in my opinion, the most powerful female force in the universe. She has four sets of twins and a ninth son called Abikú said to be an incarnation of death itself.

The following are Centella Ndoki's attributes:

Colors: All colors except black, brown
Fruit: Papaya
Herb: Caimitillo
Beverage: Aguardiente, beer
Mineral: Bronze
Animals: Guinea fowl, hens
Condiment: Eggplant
Stick: Guara
Number: 9

These are some of the most honored orishas. There are many others, but to describe all of them would require a large volume dedicated to just that, a work I may undertake in the future-R C.

CHAPTER 6

CHOMOLONGOS / IBBO / DILOGGUN COWRY SHELL DIVINATION

Diloggun, also called IBBO, is one of the foundations of ZAMBIA - PALO MONTE. It is the mouth of the Orisha. The deities eat and talk by way of the cowry shells. Only Santeria Padrinos or Palo Tatas have the authority to use this form of divination. Lucero gets 21 cowries, most other orisha 18, though in all cases only 16 are cast. The traditional way of casting, the shells is as follows:

All present must sit on the floor around a straw mat. The Tata gets the Lucero shells out, setting five aside as he says over each one, respectively, *"Ko si iku, Ko si arun, Ko si ofo, and Ko si araye"* which means "keep away death, sickness, envy, losses, and tragedy."

I assume that the Tata has already, early in the morning, said his *Mo Juba* prayers, so I won't go into it here. The taking away of the five shells is called the *Agdeye* ceremony. With the remaining 16 shells, the Tata proceeds to ask the Guardian Angel of the person being read for permission to touch the person's forehead with both hands containing cowries, naming the person saying, *"So-and-so comes before us today asking, guidance."* Lucero is then petitioned to help the individual by talking to the caster through the shells.

The shells are taken into the right hand and are gently dropped on the straw mat. The first two "throws" are considered the most important. There are 16 possibilities the shells can fall on, depending on how many fall with the natural aperture facing up. Each of these positions is called an *Oddu,* or chapter, in the diloggun corpus. All other combinations are *Omoddu,* children of the Oddu, and are obtained by combining two throws. For example, if the first throw is seven shells *(Odi)* and the second six *(Obara)* the Omoddu is *"Odibara,"* which some people simply read as a combination of Odi and Obara, but knowledgeable priests know to be a totally different chapter, just as a child of two parents is a totally different person from either of her parents, although she may resemble both.

Cowries prepared for reading are opened on the closed side, so they will have a natural opening and an artificial opening. Most Tatas learn to read only to Oddu number twelve, only the most experienced Tatas know how to read all 16 Oddus. Some houses that have grown subservient to priests of Ifa will not read beyond Oddu 12, taking the client to a *Babalawo* (Priest of Ifa) to interpret Oddus 13 through 16 if any of these come up on the first throw.

In our munanzo we always throw the shells twice at first, reading both individually as well as the Omoddu which results from the combination. We then find out whether the Oddus bring *Ire* (good fortune) or *Osogbo* (obstacles). We have some implements we use in this section of the ceremony called *Ibbo.* Traditionally, five Ibbo are used, though two are all that is really needed if one is to simplify things. The five Ibbo are: a white stone called *Otanfun,* a dark stone *(Otan Du),* a small, long shell *(Eyo),* the head of a tiny doll *(Eri Aworan),* a bone from a goat's foot or from a human hand *(Egun),* and a piece of cascarilla chalk *(Efun).*

The first question to ask with the Ibbo is whether the Oddu comes with Ire or Osogbo. The white stone and the dark stone are given to the person being read, he or she is told to gently mix the two stones, later separating one in each hand, making two fists and presenting the closed fists to the reader. The reader then throws the cowries. If a major Oddu comes up (1, 2, 3, 4, 8, 10, 12, 13, 14, 15, and 16 the reader asks for the left hand. If a minor Oddu comes up (5, 6, 7, 9, and 11), the reader asks the person being read to give him the Ibbo that he is holding in his/her right hand. If a white stone is obtained, the Oddu comes with Ire, if the dark one, with Osogbo.

Some Tatas use the white stone as Osogbo and the Cascarilla Chalk as Ire as a means of minimizing the bad fortune! The long shell is used in questions of health and/or money, the doll's head when it must be determined whether the person being read or another member of her immediate family is being alluded to. The bone is used to ask about death or the dead. Some paleros use a small cross to ask if the Ire is firm in the heavens. Using this method, a great deal of information is acquired, for each Oddu that comes up, including the ones used to determine which hand is to be opened, have something to say. At the end of the reading, it must be determined which Ibbo if any is needed to establish balance in the client or godchild's life.

The sixteen ODDU are:

1. OKANA	9. OSA
2. EYIOKO	10. OFUN
3. OGUNDA	11. OJUANI
4. IROSO	12. EYILA
5. OSHE	13. METANLA
6. OBARA	14. MERINLA
7. ODI	15. MANUNLA
8. EYEUNLE	16. MERINDILOGGUN

Firstly, let us deal with some problematic "throws."

If *Iroso Tonti* **(4-4)** comes out, the person being read may be an elder from another house come to test you, so beware of strangers that come up 4-4!

If *Ogunda Tonti* **(3-3)** comes out, immediately ask if tragedy awaits you or the person you're reading for, and if a rooster is enough to break the Oddu. If Ogunda Tonti brings Ire, wash the cowries in cold water, place them behind your door on the floor for a minute, and keep refreshing them throughout the reading, if it comes with Osogbo, leave the reading for another day and go out to look for a rooster for Ogun immediately!

If *Ofun Mafun* **(10-10)** comes up with osogbo, eight lines must be drawn behind the door with cascarilla and cocoa butter. At the end of the reading, the shells must be washed with herbs sacred to Obatala, as must the person being read.

THE IRES

Ire Aiku
Dead bring good fortune

Ire Otonowa
firm in heaven

Ire Aye
firm in the earth

Ire Elese
at the feet of an orisha
[ask which one]

Ire Lowo
by own hand

Ire Omo
through a son

Ire Eledda
through own head

Ire Enyoko
Through karma

Ire Okuni
through a man

Ire Obini
through a woman

Ire T'Olokun
through the sea

Ire Elese Egun
through a guardian spirit/
ancestor

Ire Owo
through money

Ire Ara Oko
through the countryside

Ire Elese Arugbo
through an elderly
person

Ire Ara Onu
(through the great beyond)

Ire Elese Aburo
through a brother or
godbrother

THE OSOGBOS

IKU (death)
ARUN (sickness)
EYO (envy, blood)
OFO (loss)

ONA (obstacles)
AKOBA (revolution)
FITIBO (problems)

THE ODDUS

Note: *There are good books in Spanish on the Oddu, the best being* **'Secretos de la Religion Yoruba'***. In English, the best to date is* **'Sixteen Cowries'** *by William Bascom.*

CHAPTER 7

SPELLS & FIRMAS: WORKING THE SPIRIT

The present treatise, based on the wisdom of a remarkable man, Demetrio Gomez of Guanabacoa, has not been put together with the beginner in mind. It is, in fact, a sophisticated compendium intended for the initiate. The advanced firmas (sygills) we reproduce here, from Don Demetrio's own handwritten notebooks, are filled with information the knowledgeable palero will have no trouble recognizing. None of these power signs will work for you if you have not been given a personal firma of your own. By going over the preliminary procedures involving the "how-to" of these sygills, I do not mean to talk down to our readers, whom I presume to be knowledgeable. At the same time, there are many bona fide initiates who have been cut off from their elders for any number of reasons. With this in mind, and just as a matter of refreshing some memories, I will go over the basic ceremony that, with minor adjustments, serves to empower these sygills so they may help the practitioner obtain his desired end. The following ceremony of empowerment of the sygills has been taken directly from Don Demetrio's handwrittten notebooks and is in the Mayombe tradition. As paleros you must rely heavily on your relationship with your muertos; it is your communication with your own spirit guides that will inspire you to adjust this ceremony to your particular situations and needs.

Trust your instincts, otherwise you have no business working with Palo!

1. Paint black a square piece of plywood which measures a square foot and is about one inch thick. Draw your personal firma on it using white paint or pembe chalk.

2. Prepare another piece of plywood in the same fashion. Draw the appropriate sygill you will be working with using the appropriate color paint. When in doubt, work with black and white.

3. Place both painted plywood squares on the floor next to each other, in the middle of the room or outdoor space where the working ("juego") will take place. If you've invited other paleros to participate in the juego, they should draw their firmas on pieces of brown paper bags and place them around the plywood squares. The cauldron (nganga) should rest on top of both wood sygills.

4. The officiating palero must now light a black candle and, using the wax that melts from it, he will draw three horizontal stripes of wax across each side of the blade of the knife that will be used to sacrifice the animal or animals that will be used in the working.

5. The animal is now ritually walked into the room. (if a goat or lamb, on its own feet, if a bird or small mammal, it may be carried in). As the animal's mouth and feet are ritually washed with chamba, the officiating palero recites or sings "Kiao lumbo!" "Kiao lumbo!" Kiao lumbo!"

6. The officiating palero now touches the animal's head to each male palero's genital area and female palera's breasts.

7. The officiating palero now states in a commanding voice what the purpose for the garthering is. He must be explicit, for example, he might say: "We are here to invoke Zarabanda by the power of these sygills so that our sister Mary will be blessed with a better job."

8. The officiating palero now shows the knife to the animal while softly singing "buen meme (if a goat) y a lesa kwame." This means "Good goat, you will go into a deep slumber."

9. The knife is now presented to the nganga while those present sing "meme kawida mbele kiamene ekimenga nkisi," which means "This goat's life-force will be offered to the spirits of this nganga, may they accept our sacrifice."

10. When the knife enters the animal's throat, all present sing: "Ahora si menga va corre! Menga va come, si que menga va come." (Now blood will surely run, will surely run, blood will surely run).

11. Spilling blood on a plate full of salt that had been placed there before hand, the officiating palero now sings "Fogoro yarifo, menga corre menga sangro sal la la la." Blood is, of course, poured directly on the nganga.

12. The animal is now decapitated and its severed head is placed on top of the nganga.

13. The sygills are now empowered, paleros now sing mambos and tell the spirits what must be done.

Firma Siete Rayos
TO HELP AN INMATE ACHIEVE FREEDOM

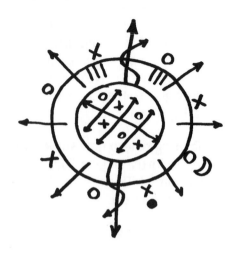

Paint this firma in four different colors. You may paint it on the ground or on a piece of cedar wood about three feet by three feet. Always paint from the center out. A white quail and a brown one must be sacrificed to Siete Rayos and left in the middle of the sygill to rot. White flour must be used to trace the inner circle, gunpowder over the outer circle. The mambo that empowers this work is the following:

Licencia agó, se va que kuenda Sambiampungo
Sambianliri, Nsambi Sururucuru,
Sambia bilongo, Siete Rayos me cutare ndian,
ndian kuenda salansanyo,
mundo garabatea,
mumbara. Licencia mi Tata, licencia to nfunbi,
licencia to ndianbe, licencia cuadrilla Congo,
licencia Cuatro Vientos, licencia Tango,
lisencia nsulu, licencia ntoto, licencia
Mama Nsala, Que va kuenda bajo ntoto.
Sala maleko, maleko sala.

FIRMA SIETE RAYOS
TO EMPOWER A HOUSE AND
MAKE THE TATA STRONG AND HEALTHY

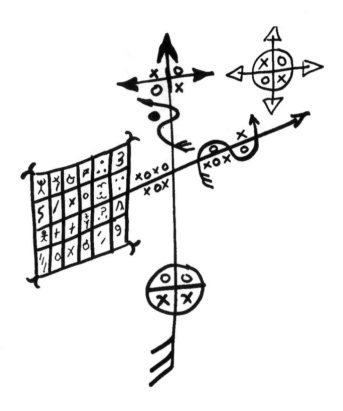

Draw this firma in front of the main nganga using cascarilla, pembe, or chalk. A ram, two white quails, two brown quails, two white roosters, and two tortoises must be sacrificed to Lucero and the nganga. Add red wine, dry white wine, chamba, cigar smoke, twenty-one little piles of gunpowder, and all of the main firmas of the house written on parchment.

Zarabanda Firma
TO OBTAIN MATERIAL WEALTH

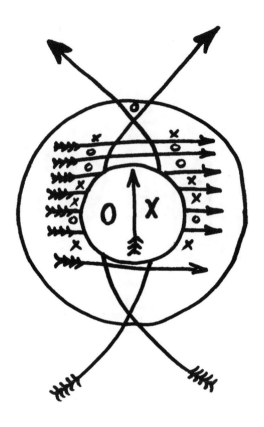

Sacrificial animals needed: two black roosters which must be passed over the person for whom the money work is being performed, the roosters are then killed without decapitating them, their bodies left on the nganga for twenty-four hours.

Zarabanda Firma
TO EXORCISE EVIL SPIRITS

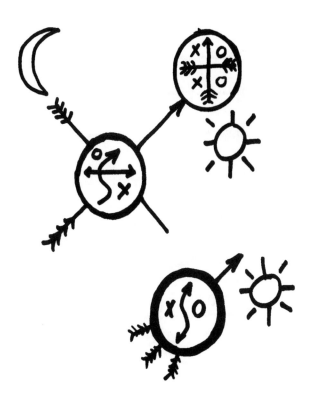

Draw firma with pembe or cascarilla on the floor in front of nganga, person to be cleansed should step on firma barefooted. Tata or Yayi now passes two roosters over person, killing them without decapitating them, sprinkling some blood on the person's bare feet, offering the rest of the blood to the nganga. Person being cleansed should erase firma with his/her feet. As the firma dissapears, so does the trouble-causing ghosts.

83

Zarabanda Firma
FOR PERMANENT PROTECTION

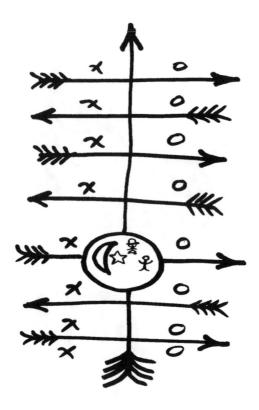

This firma should be painted in the nso, the temple where the person who seeks protection keeps his/her nganga. I have made this firma a permanent part of the decoration of my munanso. It requires the sacrifice of two guinea fowl, a black rooster, and a quail.

Zarabanda Firma
TO MAKE AN AMULET
THAT MAKES ONE INVISIBLE TO THE POLICE

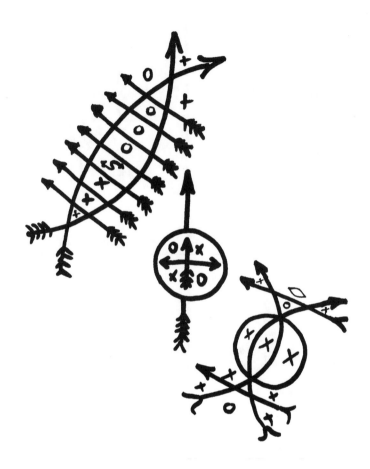

Draw this firma in parchment or a piece of brown paper bag. Place on top of nganga, sacrifice two black pigeons, a red rooster, and two white quails. Make sure some of the blood of each animal reaches the paper. Afterwards, fold paper and place inside small leather bag along with a hummingbird heart. Carry amulet (makuto) with you at all times.

85

SOME SIMPLE FIRMAS
DEPICTING THE NKISIS

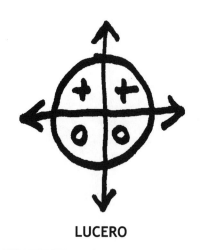

LUCERO

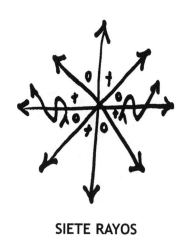

SIETE RAYOS

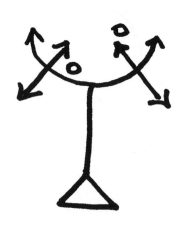
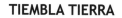

TIEMBLA TIERRA

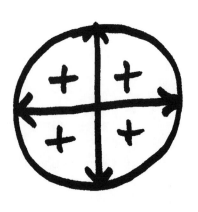

ZARABANDA

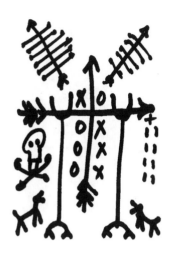

PATA EN LLAGA

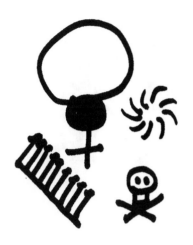

CENTELLA NDOKI

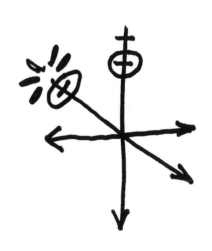

MAMA CHOLA
WANGA

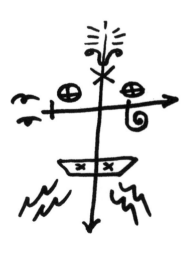

MAMA KALUNGA

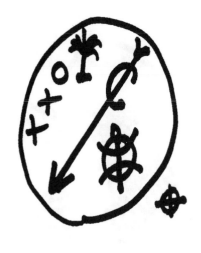

NGURUFINDA

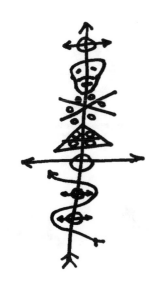

NFUIRI

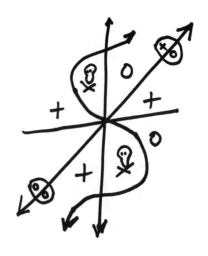

FIRMA TO WORK WITH GUNPOWDER

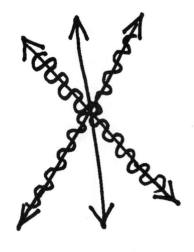

**MAMA KENGUE
AS CREATOR OF THE UNIVERSE**

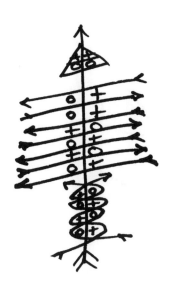

BALAUNDE

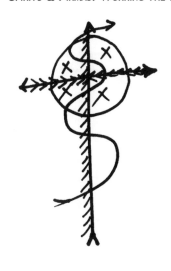

KALUNGA

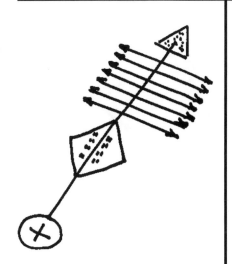

SIETE RAYOS
For Winning Battles

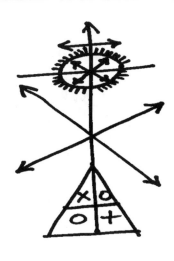

LUCERO

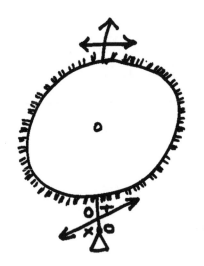

MAMAKENGUE

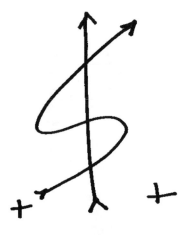

NKUYO ABRE CAMINOS
Always Opens Roads!
Used to Open Ceremony

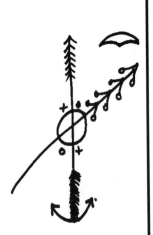

MAMA SHOLA

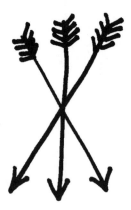

NKUYO LUCERO
Used to close
ceremonies

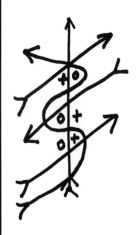

NKUYO

Some simple Palo ideographs

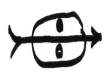

Malongo *(nature)*

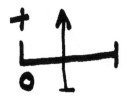

Ngo *(government)*

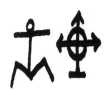

Mama Nganga *(godmother)*

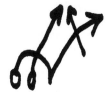

Vititi *(view; look)*

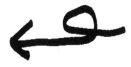

Kuenda *(go)*

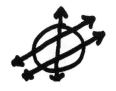

Pele-fula *(life)*

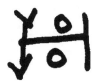

Munanzo *(house)*

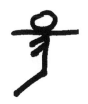

Ndumba *(woman)*

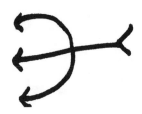

Place

Trust

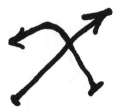

Everything

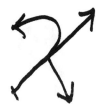

Guardian

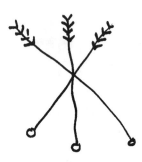

Kimbasa
Draw this firma inside
comunion bowl from where
all present will drink.

Ngueyo *(brother)*

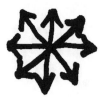

Bakonfula *(assistant Tata)*

Mayimbe *(vulture)*

Ensila *(road)*

Sunsundamba *(owl)*

Wansa *(river)*

Ntangu *(sun)*

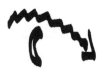

Kalunga *(sea)*

Eyioko *(snake)*

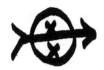

Nganga

Nsulo *(heaven)*

Spring

Lango nsulo *(rain)*

Omalembe *(pain)*

Watoko *(young man)*

Meji *(twins)*

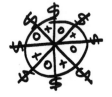

Yimbula *(party)*

Tata ngumbe *(dead father)*

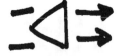

Tribe

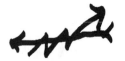

"before"

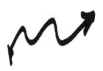

"after"

Ngonda *(crescent moon)*

CHAPTER 8

BATHS, SPELLS
AND OTHER WORKS

Palo's reputation for being "evil," "dark" or "black magic" comes from a misunderstanding of the forces that move the world. Zambia's all-encompassing energy is expressed in creation as expanding and contracting forces, the yin-yang of Taoism. Paleros work with both currents, ndoki and nsanbi. Ndoki, the negative manifestation of being, is the aspect of divinity that acts as the punishment for wrongdoers: "karma". Ndoki is dark, lunar, hidden, fluid, and primal, prima facie, ndoki appears to be evil. Ndoki is identified with the contracting aspect of the cosmos, with implosion, destruction, death and disease. Nsanbi is the positive manifestation of being. Nsanbi is bright, solar, exposed, solid, and developed. Nsanbi is identified with goodness; with the expanding cosmos, with life, birth, growth and healing. In reality, ndoki cannot exist without nsanbi and vice versa. Imagine an organism constantly inhaling without ever exhaling, it would explode! When Paleros work with ndoki, therefore, they must be extremely careful not to incur the wrath of the Lords of Karma. Only very seasoned and well-balanced practitioners should work with the forces of ndoki. Less experienced Paleros may seriously imperil their spiritual development as well as those of their clients and godchildren if they misuse the power of ndoki.

FOR GOOD LUCK

• The basic "good luck" bath is prepared with white lillies, adding its petals to your bathwater. Light a candle to Tiembla-Tierra while you are taking the bath. Do it eight Thursdays in a row.

• Another bath designed to attract good vibrations consists of adding three bay leaves to your bathwater, along with seven different perfumes/colognes. Repeat seven times, once per week.

• If you find signs of a work against you outside your home, such as a dead chicken or a bunch of bananas etc. urinate on the work, then discard it. If in your household there's a young boy (girls' urine is not thought proper, for some reason), then let him urinate on it, for an innocent child's urine is a more powerful spiritual cleanser than holy water blessed by the Pope. In fact, to ensure the spiritual integrity of your home, add a couple of drops of a child's urine as well as some holy water from a Catholic, Orthodox, or High Episcopalian Church to the water you use to clean your home's floors.

TO ATTRACT LOVERS

• Fill a pail half-way with water, add to it a splash of apple-blossom cologne, five drops of honey, and some lillies. Immediately after you take a shower, pour the previously-prepared pail on your body from the neck down. Do this three Wednesdays or Fridays in a row. Add parsley to the ingredients and it becomes a money-drawing bath as well.

• Another bath to attract a lover is made by filling a pail 3/4 of the way with water, adding to it parsley, petals from five carnations, five drops of honey, a white rose (petals only), and a splash of Florida Water. Pour pail on your body from the neck down—make sure your genitals get plenty! Repeat bath five Wednesdays or Fridays in a row.

• *To make a man you know fall in love with you* (this spell does not work on a woman) steal one of his handkerchiefs, pass it all over your naked body and leave it in as intimate a part of your body as you can for twenty-four hours. If you can get hairs from him, mix them with your own hair and burn them in the flame of a seven-day white candle. Look at the candle's flame intently, visualizing the man's face. When his features appear clear in your mind's eye, the spell has been successful.

• Adding a couple of drops of your menstrual blood to coffee you make for your loved one makes him fall madly in love with you; he will not be able to think of anybody else.

• *To make a loved one come back after he has left you,* take a pumpkin and hollow it out, keeping the top as a lid. Take five nails from the feet of a rooster and put them inside the hollowed pumpkin, adding an egg, marjoram, the name of the loved one written on parchment paper and any personal item you may have of the person you want back. Spit inside the pumpkin three times, then close the pumpkin using the lid. Place the pumpkin next to Mama Chola Wanga for five days, then offer it to the river along with five pennies. Your stray lover will come back within twenty-one days.

MONEY-DRAWING BATHS AND WORKS

• In a bathtub full of warm water, pour five cups of milk, five bunches of curly parsley, and five drops of honey. Bathe for at least twenty minutes asking Mama Chola Wanga to bless you with money.

• *To attract business,* clean the doorway of your place with parsley, cinnamon, and honey in water. Afterward, spread some cornmeal around.

• When writing a letter asking for money, pass some cascarilla over the paper in which you are to write the letter before setting pen to paper.

HEALING HERBS

• Boiled leaves, stems, and bark of myrtle make a great skin cleanser.

• Soursop leaves should be boiled and applied directly to the side of the face that is affected by neuralgia.

• Linden flowers and leaves make a great calming tea for nervous or easily excited people.

• Chamomille tea is good to settle an upset stomach and as a natural shampoo for the hair.

• Mango seeds, ground to a powder and mixed with water make a first-rate disinfectant.

SEPARATING SPELLS

• *To bring serious discord to a home*, take nine peony seeds, black pepper, and leaves from a peanut plant, burn all to a crisp. Blow the resulting ashes on the door of the people you want to see fighting among each other.

• *To separate a couple*, take seven pumpkin leaves, mix with twenty-one kernels of black pepper, grind to a powder, blow on door of targeted couple.

• *To keep someone away,* take dirt from the bottom of a nganga, seeds from three okras, dirt from a crossroads, and the name of the person you want far. Put these things in a bottle weighted so that it goes to the bottom of a river, where you must throw it at twelve midnight.

MORE ON HERBS AND PLANTS

Although many of the herbs used in Palo may be difficult to find in some areas, there are enough common plants available in most places to honor each orisha. The following are certain fairly common plants and herbs associated with the following deities.

LUCERO
Asafetida
Chili Pepper Grass
Black Eyed Pea Leaves

SIETE RAYOS
Bananas
Palm fronds
China berry

TIEMBLA TIERRA
Lillies
Cotton
Almond
Avocado leaves
Coffee
Guava
Dried rosebuds

MADRE DE AGUA
Indigo
Seaweed
Purple basil
Bell pepper
Lotus
Sponge
(not a plant, but functions as one)
Driftwood

PATA EN LLAGA
Ivy
Myrtle
ginger

ZARABANDA
Cayenne pepper
Black pepper
Oak leaves

MAMA CHOLA WANGA	CENTELLA NDOKI
Fern, Orange blossom	Camphor
Papaya, Anise	Cypress
Witch hazel, Vervain	All beans
Purple grapes	Peanut
Roses	Hemp
Coriander	Rose of Jericho *(stem only)*

SECRETS OF ANDRES PETIT:

One of Don Demetrio's most fabulous teachers was Andres Petit, a ceremonial magician whose powers, in my opinion, were greater than Eliphas Levi's and possibly equal to Aleister Crowley's. Petit was a lay member of the order of the Friars Minors (Franciscans) of the Roman Catholic Church, called a "terciary" member. He was familiar with European grimoires, which he read in Latin. But his area of greatest expertise was in African-derived religions. He became infamous (or beloved, depending on who you ask) when in 1863 he initiated the first white men to the ultra-secret magical Abakua society, which in turn opened the doors of all of the other Afro-Cuban religious expressions to whites and mulattoes. Hated by blacks who accused him of "selling out our power for eighty ounces of silver" because of what he did, his action nevertheless helped preserve Afro-Cuban religions. Andres Petit's motives for initiating non-blacks was not personal gain, in fact, he had taken vows of poverty and although he dressed in exquisite Savile row suits, he wore sandals and used all of his money to help those less fortunate. He is said to have bought freedom for hundreds of slaves.

When Petit's faction of Abakua was threatened by other factions who resented the inclusion of non-blacks, Petit organized his Palo godchildren into a duly-instituted religious organization, La Regla Kimbisa del Santo Cristo del Buen Viaje, with the express purpose of forming a magical army against any attack. Petit wrote all the articles, by-laws, rituals, and hierarchical structures of the order.

The Kimbisa faction of Palo, as his branch became known, has the most clearly delneated rules and regulations of any Congo-Cuban (Palo) denomination. Following are some workings taken from some of Tata Quien Vence's (Petit's) unpublished journals.

INSPIRATION: WORKING WITH THE KIMBISA FIRMAS

Before actually working with any of the following firmas, say the welcoming prayer which follows, either in its original Spanish, or in my translation.

>*"Inspiracion divina, bienvenido seas a este templo al que con los fluidos poderosos del Padre nos trae una comunicacion a nosotros los de este plano tierra, Asi como San Juan Nepomuceno desato su lengua., que la tuya se desate, como to manda la Santa Obediencia, para que men mboba to to muana"*

>*"Divine Inspiration, I bid you welcome to this temple to which, with the powerful vibrations of the Father, you bring us on this earthly plane communications. Just as St. John Nepomucene untied his tongue, may yours be untied, as Holy Obedience demands, so that all brethren may benefit."*

KIMBISA PRAYER TO PREVENT PSYCHIC ATTACKS

>*Oh most Holy Nkisi, Sacrament of the Altar, God of Nature, Three Persons and One True Essence, under the protection of the Institution of the Holy Christ of the Pleasant Journey, take my thoughts from Ntoto to Nsukururu, where my Holy Guardian Angels will listen to them and grant me protection.*

(continued)

Oh Kongo Kimbisa Batalla Holy Christ of the Pleasant Journey, take away, restrict, and put down any and all dibolical act, bad thought, malembe from the living or the dead, evil eye, bad words, and make me kin to the Holy Trinity in times of pain of the body and the soul. Protect me while I sleep and receive and keep my spirit till I wake, giving it instructions. For my salvation with the Holy Trinity of the Holy Christ of the Pleasant Journey which has Overcome, Overcomes, and will Overcome, Amen. (Light a white candle and place a glass full of water next to it)

WORK TO MAKE SOMEONE LOVE YOU

1. Draw firma (see page 98) using yellow pembe or yellow paint on flat ground.

2.
   Light yellow candle dressed with cinnamon and honey.

3.
   Say following prayer:

   "Chola cholanwere Chola Ntoche ntoche alamutanche Cholan were alagongue ndo Kinkelele tonche Aweben Chola Vamo a bombi alabomeiton tonche Nkanu Kimbangara Kimbangara Mbonguere oniseto moniseto."

4.
   To a cup of water, add the white of an egg and some Mercury. Let the light of the sun hit it, and say: "Just as mercury is never still may_____ never be able to rest until (s)he comes to me."

5.
   Leave cup in middle of firma for five days, then remove, wipe out firma, and throw cup with contents in a river along with five pennies. Your intended will come to you within 21 days.

FIRMA MAMA CHOLA
TO FIND A LOVER

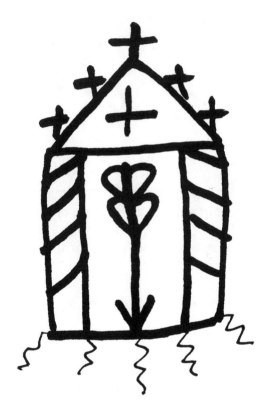

MAMA CHOLA EBOLA WANGA (KIMBISA)

KIMBISA DEFENSIVE ACTION TO SEND BACK EVIL
USING ST. BARBARA'S FIRMA

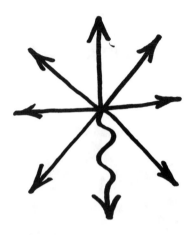

1. Use cascarilla to draw firma on the ground.

2. Alternate three white and three red finger candles, putting one at the point of each straight arrow of the firma, and place a black one alt the point of the one wiggly arrow. Widdershins, starting on the arrow immediately to the left of the wiggly arrow, light each candle.

3. Say the following prayer while standing by the black candle.

   "Bendito Babd, Santa Barbara bendita Subitera yen yen Yerbere yebere yebete Yambe yambe yambe Ba ya mo Dame una muna como Tata Kenyen kisa sinamba Boma karire Mboma Nsasi kina mututu yeta yeta Muana longo. Pluma de cotorra colord Garabata garabatd Kimbisa yoma kimbisa Verifuasi hay, Congo!"

4. Snuff out candles, erase firma with your right hand using a clockwise motion. Place all remains of candles in a bag with seven pennies, deposit by a large tree in a park or wooded area.

JUEGO DE BALUANDE PARA SUERTE Y DINERO
(WORKING FOR GOOD LUCK AND MONEY)

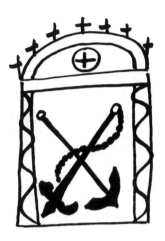

1. Using cascarilla, draw firma on the ground, next to your nganga (if you do not have one, next to a machete)

2. Arrange 7 bunches of parsley, 7 heads of lettuce, and 7 bunches of water-cress in front of firma.

3. Light a white candle and say the following prayer:

    Gan gan gan Baluande to Kongo yero Gan gan gan guimbo kalunguera Nkelele munanganga nkimbo kalungera Simba muana nsun nsusu Muana ganga kualinkintaya Bobelende Bobelende Bobelende Nlogue nlogue ae! Kewande quiere Kalunga ye ye ye to mule Uria nguimbo kalunguera Nguimbo lalunguera Mama Tete Uria niongue nlongue nlongue lunguan fula gangule Aguelie su mare pobrecito criollo.

4. Light a small mound of fula on the tip of a machete.

5. Take off clothes and rub herbs all over your body.

6. Gather all remnants and put on a plastic bag, leave by a prosperous bank at midnight.

"JUEGO SAN PEDRO" (WORKING WITH ST. PETER) FOR PROTECTION.

From the unpublished journals of Andres Petit, founder of the Kimbisa faction of Palo.

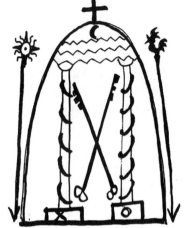

1. Using cascarilla, draw a circle large enough so that all present can stand inside it, the one person receiving the blessing (being worked on) kneeling in the middle.

2. On a white piece of wood at least 3' by 3'that is lying in the middle of the circle, draw the firma of St. Joseph using fula.

3. The presiding Palero now asks each participant *"Quien Kuenda?"* to which each must respond with his or her initiation name and steps inside circle, facing the center. If any present, other than the person being worked on, does not have a palo initiation name, he or she has to remain outside the circle.

4. The person receiving the blessing now kneels in the middle, next to the firma. The presiding Palero puts one hand on the person's head while with the other he holds a white lit candle. An assistant may hold a paper with the invocation to St. Peter written on it so the presiding Palero can read it, if he doesn't know it by heart.

5. The presiding Palero, or a designated second, now says the invocation to St. Peter out loud.

"*Va con licencia Nganga Nsila*
Va con licencia Nganga Nkisa
Va con licencia Palo Monte
Va con licencia Nsusu Susundamba
Va con licencia Nsusu Mayimbe
Va con licencia Ntoto Cuatro Vientos
Va con licencia Ntoto Gifri
Va con licencia Plaza Lirio
Va con licencia Mama Kiyumba
Va con licencia to to Moana Nsambia Kien Vence   Va
nkuti nkuyo que va uria Malafo y nsunga le de fuerza
y poder sobrenatural al nkisa sobre sus enemigos
visibles a invisibles.

6. The presiding Palero, standing behind the kneeling person, now blows smoke on both of his/her shoulders, and sprays rum from his mouth on the back of the person's neck.

7. The person is helped to his or her feet, the fula that had formed the firma is gathered and divided in two piles. One is given to the person being worked on to add to his or her next bath. The other half is put on the tip of a machete and lighted by the presiding Palero.

8. The Palero now asks person he has helped to erase the circle in a counter-clockwise fashion using his/her naked foot.

9. Chomolongos or coconuts are consulted to make sure all went well. If the answer is no, usually more rum, more cigar smoke, or some water, honey, or molassess must be presented to St. Peter. The Palero will ask, "does St. Peter want more rum?" etc., until he receives a positive answer.

WORKING WITH LUNGAMBE
TO MAKE BUSINESS PROSPER

1. Using palm oil, draw Lungambe's firma behind door of bathroom in the business that is to be blessed, then light a green candle to Lungambe.

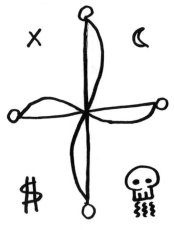

2. Sing or recite following mambo

> *Lungambe no quiere a nadie*
> *Lungambe mato a su madre*
> *Lungambe mato a su padre*
> *Lungambe no tiene amigo*
> *Lungambe es gangulero*
> *Lungambe los malos palos*
> *Lungambe to tronco e'ceiba*
> *Lungambe to tata nfunbe Lungambe!*

3. In a juicer, make some starfruit juice using four fruits. Add a cup of red wine to it, smoked jutia, smoked fish, honey, and water. Pour some of the liquid in front of your business, save the rest.

4. Add flour to remaining liquid until it has consistency of hard clay, make two balls, give one to Nkuyo so that whoever means you harm gets f----d up, and the other to Lungambe so that much money comes to the business.

CLEANSING WITH CENTELLA

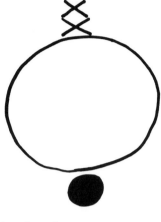

1. Draw firma inside an empty cauldron, using with cascarilla.

2. Add an egg, nine handkerchiefs (each a different color), and four remnants of four candles (unlit).

3. Sacrifice a chick to the work.

4. Recite the following prayer:

   Temporal tumba palo como no tumba ojo.
   Eh! vamo alla Batalla Sierite la Loma
   No digo Madiata Guiaguo
   Barikoso dayo lindero cimbra ciguaraya
   Macreto bilongo.

5. Light a small pile of fula.

6. Take egg out of cauldron and throw high outside, letting it break as it falls.

7. Remaining stuff in cauldron can be saved for future works with Centella.

CHAPTER 9

SOME IMPORTANT
PRAYERS & MAMBOS

These most important of all Palo incantations or mambos, some published for the first time ever, are considered extremely important to the practice of Palo, the heart and soul of the sacrificial ceremonies. They are sung in a creolized Spanish called "Bozal." The reason I am not translating the mambos into English is that their content is either nonsensical or so abstract as to not make sense grammatically speaking. What the Palo Masters who composed these mambos were looking for was not cohesive oratory, but a confluence of vocals and consonants that when emitted at certain ceremonial occassions would cause the veil that separates the world of the unseen from the material world to be temporarily lifted.

Take the mambo *"Porque gallina no planta gallo, porque"* as an example. These lyrics mean "Because hen doesn't plant rooster, because." See what I mean? The important thing is to try to sing these mambos as closely as possible to the way they are written, without worrying about what they mean.

When the Tata inserts the sacrificial knife in the throat of an animal, all present should sing the following:

> *Meme (or ensuso if its a rooster, etc.) kabwinda*
> *embele kiamene*
> *eki menga nkisi*

When the Tata's helper lifts the animal up, allowing its blood to flow on the prenda, all members present must sing as follows:

> *Ahora si menga va corre, como corre*
> *Ahora si menga va corre, si señó*
> *Ahora si menga va corre*

When feeding other implements after nganga and Lucero have received the first offering, the following mambo is intoned:

> *Fogoro yarifo*
> *menga corre menga*
> *Fogoro yarifo*

At this time a plate or dish made out of half a gourd containing some salt is placed under the animal's throat to collect its remaining blood, while this is going on, all present will sing:

> *Sangra sala lai la lai la,*
> *lai la lai la, lai la lai la.*

OTHER ESSENTIAL PRAYERS

ENTERING THE NSO (PRESENCE OF THE NGANGA)

> *Burunkisa nganga*
> *Nguangara nkunia*
> *Munanfua monunkuame*
> *Tata ndibilongo tuyembere*

OPENING PRAYER

Guiriko nganga
Mbonda Tata Nganga Monte Mayombe
Kuenda Camposanto Medianoche
Andres Petit Zarabanda Mata Mundele
Licencia Zambia
Zambia arriba, Zambia abajo,
Zambia en lo cuatro costao
Licencia Lucero Tata Ndoki
Licencia Ntango, Licencia Mposi
Licencia Nsambi, Licencia Ndoki
Licencia Ntoto, Licencia Nsulo
Licencia Kalunga, Licencia Kunalemba
Licencia Kunasinda, Licencia Kunafinda
Licencia Nfunbi vititi bacheche
Nfunbi vititi guariguari
Licencia to lo nfunbi
Guiriko nganga
Somo o no somo?
SOMO!

OATH OF LOYALTY / CREDE

Tendundu
Kienpunguele
Mani masango
Nsilan banza
mandie
Sese mandie
Bikan bioko
Bigan diame
Ndilicuame
Nsambi ndiganga!

PRAYER FOR THE RAZOR BLADE

Kabanga Tengue
Pian kilanga
Tala moko
Nganga nkisa
Nkita mulanga
Ngungu nsanguila
Sogulo basula
Kuenda muini
Mbanzo
Nmusi naba
Nguenguere

Prayer to Sacrifice a Goat
(To be whispered in its ear and nose)

Turunbanguele!
Turunbanguele!
Turunbanguele!
Turunbanguele!
Turunbanguele!
Turunbanguele!
Turunbanguele!

Prayer to Sacrifice a Turtle or a Tortoise
(Never use a knife, use a pointed stone instead)

Nfuru
Batiakitatio
Fotankualo

Prayer to Sacrifice a Duck

Baluande kiambi ko
Kiamfunda Kalunga
Kiambonga nsusu Suakara!
(its head is then placed by its side)

Salutation of the Nganga

Zambia mpungi, vititi losa
tava sili, mono panibele
Machuco Kongo, Lunguanda buengue.

"PORQUE"

Guia. - Porque Gallina, no siembra Gallo . . . . . . Porque.
Coro. - Porque Gallina, no siembra Gallo . . . . . . Porque.
Guia. - A Chapear Cantero.
Coro. - Porque Gallina, no siembra Gallo . . . . . . Porque.
Guia. - A Chapear Cantero.
Coro. - Porque Gallina, no siembra Gallo . . . . . . Porque.
Guia. - A Chapear Cantero.
Coro. - Porque Gallina, no siembra Gallo . . . . . . Porque.
Guia. - Porque Gallina, no siembra Gallo . . . . . . Porque.
Coro. - Porque Gallina, no siembra Gallo . . . . . . Porque.
Guia. - A Chapear Cantero.
Coro. - Porque Gallina, no siembra Gallo . . . . . . Porque.
Guia. - A Chapear Cantero.
Coro. - Porque Gallina, no siembra Gallo . . . . . . Porque.
Guia. - A Chapear Cantero.
Coro. - Porque Gallina, no siembra Gallo . . . . . . Porque.
Guia. - A Chapear Cantero.
Coro. - Porque Gallina, no siembra Gallo . . . . . . Porque.
Guia. - A Chapear Cantero.
Coro. - Porque Gallina, no siembra Gallo . . . . . . Porque.
Guia. - A Chapear Cantero.
Coro. - Porque Gallina, no siembra Gallo . . . . . . Porque.
Guia. - Mambe.
Coro. - Dios.
Guia. - Mambe.
Coro. - Dios.
Guia. - Mambe.
Coro. - Dios.

"ENDUNDO"

Coro. - Endundo, Endundo.
Guia. - Misma Palma son Endundo.
Coro. - Endundo, Endundo.
Guia. - Mismo Toto, son Endundo.
Coro. - Endundo, Endundo.
Guia. - Mismo Fumbi, son
Endundo.
Coro. - Endundo, Endundo.
Guia. - Misma Nganga, son
Endundo.
Coro. - Endundo, Endundo.
Guia. - Misma Tierra, son
Endundo.
Coro. - Endundo, Endundo.
Guia. - Mismo Palo, son Endundo.
Coro. - Endundo, Endundo.
Guia. - Misma Kinyumba, son
Endundo.
Coro. - Endundo, Endundo.

Guia. - Mambe.
Coro. - Dios.
Guia. - Mambe.
Coro. - Dios.
Guia. - Mambe.
Coro. - Dios.

"BUENAS NOCHES"

Coro.- Buenas noches, buenas
noches,
Guia.- Buenas noches mi Lucerito,
Buenas noches, buenas noches,
Buenas mi Tiembla-Tierra,
Buenas noches, buenas noches,
Buenas noches, mi 7 Rayos,
Buenas noches, buenas noches,
Buenas noches mi Madre de Agua,
Buenas noches, buenas noches,
Buenas noches mi Sholan
Guengue,
Buenas noches, buenas noches,
Buenas noches, mi Pata en Llaga,
Buenas noches, buenas noches,
Buenas noches mi Centellita,.
Buenas noches, buenas noches,
Buenas noches mi Zarabanda,
Buenas noches, buenas noches,
Buenas noches tenga mi Nganga,
Buenas noches, buenas noches,
Buenas noches tenga mi palo,
Buenas noches, buenas noches,
Buenas noches mi Madre Ceiba,
Buenas noches, buenas noches,
Buenas noches a Limpia Piso,
Buenas noches, buenas noches,
Buenas noches mi sigue rastro,
Buenas noches, buenas noches,
Buenas noches a Mayordomo,
Buenas noches, buenas noches,
Buenas noches a to lo Empaca,
Buenas noches, buenas noches,
Buenas noches a la Cuadrilla,
Buenas noches, buenas noches,
Buenas noches a Manzanero,
Buenas noches, buenas noches,

"LUMBE, LUMBE, LUMBE"

Lumbe, lumbe, lumbe, lumbe la cueva en Nganga,
Si Lucerito, tá cere cere,
Coro. - Palo Kindiambo ace ague,
Guia. - Lumbe, lumbe, lumbe, lumbe la cueva en Nganga,
Tiembla-Tierra, tá cere cere,
Palo Kindiambo ace ague,
Lumbe, lumbe, lumbe, lumbe la cueva en Nganga,
Si 7 Rayos tá cere cere,
Palo Kindiambo ace ague,
Lumbe, lumbe, lumbe, lumbe la cueva en Nganga,
Si Madre de Aqua tá cere cere,
Palo Kindiambo acece ague,
Lumbe, lumbe, lumbe, lumbe la cueva en Nganga,
Si Sholán Guengue tá cere cere,
Palo Kindiambo acece ague,
Lumbe, lumbe, lumbe, lumbe la cueva en Nganga,
Si Pata en Llaga, tá cere cere,
Palo Kindiambo acece ague,
Lumbe, lumbe, lumbe, lumbe la cueva en Nganga,
Si Centellita tá cere cere,
Palo Kindiambo acece ague,
Lumbe, lumbe, lumbe, lumbe la cueva en Nganga,
Si Zarabanda tá cere cere,
Palo Kindiambo acece ague,
Lumbe, lumbe, lumbe, lumbe la cueva en Nganga,
Si la Nganga, tá cere cere,
Palo Kindiambo acece ague,
Lumbe, lumbe, lumbe, lumbe la cueva en Ngnnga,
Si Madre Ceiba, tá cere cere,
Palo Kindiambo acece ague,
Lumbe, lumbe, lumbe, lumbe la cueva en Nganga,
Si la cuadrilla, tá cere cere,
Palo Kindiambo acece ague,
Lumbe, lumbe, lumbe, lumbe la cueva en Nganga,
Si limpia piso, cere cere,
Palo Kindiambo acece ague,
Lumbe, lumbe, lumbe, lumbe la cueva en Nganga,
Si Lucerito, tá cere cere.

"DEBAJO DEL LAUREL"

Debajo del Laurel, yo tengo mi confianza,
Yo tengo mi confianza, yo tengo mi confianza,
Coro. - Debajo del Laurel, yo tengo mi confianza,
Guia. - Lucero es mi confianza, Lucero es mi confianza,
Debajo del Laurel, yo tengo mi confianza,
Tiembla-Tierra, es mi confianza, Tiembla-Tierra es mi confianza,
Debajo del Laurel, yo tengo mi confianza,
7 Rayos es mi confianza, 7 Rayos es mi conflanza,
Debajo del Laurel, yo tengo mi confianza,
Madre de Agua es mi confianza, Madre de Agua es mi confianza,
Debajo del Laurel, yo tengo mi confianza,
Sholán Guengue es mi confianza, Sholán Guengue es mi confianza, Debajo
del Laurel, yo tengo mi confianza,
Pata en Llaga es mi confianza, Pata en Llaga es mi confianza,
Debajo del Laurel, yo tengo mi confianza,
Centella es mi confianza, Centella es mi confianza,
Debajo del Laurel, yo tengo mi confianza,
Zarabanda es mi confianza, Zarabanda es mi confianza,
Debajo del Laurel, yo tengo mi confianza, .
Tata en Nganga es mi confianza, Tata en Nganga es mi confianza, Debajo del
Laurel, yo tengo mi conflanza,
Palo en Nganga es mi confianza, Palo en Nganga es mi confianza,
Debajo del Laurel, yo tengo mi confianza,
Viento en Ceiba, es mi confianza, Viento en Ceiba, es mi confianza,
Debajo del Laurel, yo tengo mi confianza,
Manzanero es mi confianza, Manzanero es mi confianza,
Debajo del Laurel, yo tengo mi conflanza,
Limpia Piso es mi confianza, Limpia Piso es mi confianza,
Debajo del Laurel; yo tengo mi conflanza,
Sigue Rastro es mi confianza, Sigue Rastro es mi confianza,
Debajo del Laurel, yo tengo mi confianza,
El Mayordomo es mi confianza, El Mayordomo es mi confianza,
Debajo del Laurel; yo tengo mi conflanza,
La cuadrilla es mi confianza, La cuadrilla es mi confianza,
Debajo del Laurel, yo tengo mi confianza,
Lucero es mi confianza, Lucero es mi confianza,
Debajo del Laurel; yo tengo mi conflanza,
Mambe (Dios) Mambe (Dios) Mambe (Dios).

"AHORA VERÁN, AHORA VERÁN…"

Guia. - Ahora verán, ahora verán,
Repite el coro. - A Lucerito en la Palma, ahora verán,
Ahora verán, ahora verán,
A Tiembla-Tierra en la Palma, ahora verán,
Ahora verán, ahora verán,
A 7 Rayos en la Palma, ahora verán,
Ahora verán, ahora verán,
A Madre de Agua en la Palma,
Ahora verán, ahora verán,
A Sholán Guengue, en la Palma, ahora verán,
Ahora verán, ahora verán,
A Pata en Llaga, en la Palma, ahora verán,
Ahora verán, ahora verán,
A Centellita en la Palma, ahora verán,
Ahora verán, ahora verán,
A Zarabanda en la Palma, ahora verán,
Ahora verán, ahora verán,
Al Tata en Nganga en la Palma, ahora verán,
Ahora verán, ahora verán,
A Viento en Ceiba en la Palma, ahora verán,
Ahora verán, ahora verán,
A sigue rastro, en la Palma, ahora verán,
Ahora verán, ahora verán,
A Manzanero en la Palma, ahora verán,
Ahora verán, ahora verán,
A Limpia Piso en la Palma, ahora verán,
Ahora verán, ahora verán,
Al Mayordomo en la Palma, ahora verán,
Ahora verán, ahora verán,
A1 Padrino en la Palma, ahora verán,
Ahora verán, ahora verán,
A to lo empaca en la Palma, ahora verán,
Ahora verán, ahora verán,
A la cuadrilla en la Palma, ahora verán,
Ahora verán, ahora verán,
A Lucerito en la Palma, ahora verán,
Mambe (Dios), Mambe (Dios), Mambe (Dios).

"PA QUE TU ME LLAMAS"

Coro. - Si tú no me conoces pá qué me llamas,
Guia. - Pa qué tú me llamas, pá qué tú me llamas,
Yo soy Lucerito, pá qué tú me llamas,
Coro. - Si to no me conoces pá qué tú me llamas,
Guia. - Yo soy Tiembla-Tierra, pá qué tú me llamas,
Si tú no me conoces pá qué tú me llamas,
Yo soy 7 Rayos, pá qué tú me llamas,
Si tú no me conoces pá qué tú me llamas,
Yo soy Madre de Agua, pá qué tú me llamas,
Si tú no me conoces pá qué tú me llamas,
Yo soy Sholán Guengue, pá qué tú me llamas,
Si tú no me conoces pá qué tú me llamas,
Yo soy Pata en Llaga, pá qué tú me llamas,
Si tú no me conoces pá qué tú me llamas,
Yo soy Centellita, pá qué tú me llamas,
Si tú no me conoces pá qué tú me llamas,
Yo soy Zarabanda, pá qué tú me llamas,
Si tú no me conoces pá qué tú me llamas,
Yo soy Palo en Nganga, pá qué tú me llamas,
Si tú no me conoces pá qué tú me llamas,
Yo soy Tata en Nganga, pá qué tú me llamas,
Si tú no me conoces pá qué tú me llamas,
Yo soy Viento en Ceiba, pá qué tú me llamas,
Si tú no me conoces pá qué tú me llamas,
Yo soy Manzanero, pá qué tú me llamas,
Si tú no me conoces pá qué tú me llamas,
Yo soy Limpia piso, pá qué tú me llamas,
Si tú no me conoces pá qué tú me llamas,
Yo soy Mayordomo, pá qué tú me llamas,
Si tú no me conoces pá qué tú me llamas,
Yo soy Sigue Rastro, pá qué tú me llamas,
Si tú no me conoces pá qué tú me llamas,
Yo soy Palo en Nganga, pá qué tú me llamas,
Si tú no me conoces pá qué tú me llamas,
Yo soy Madre Ceiba, pá qué tú me llamas,
Si tú no me conoces pá qué tú me llamas,
Yo soy Lucerito, pá qué tú me llamas,
Coro. - Si tú no me conoces pá qué tú me llamas,
Guia. - Mambe (Dios), Mambe (Dios), Mambe (Dios).

"NGANGULERO"

Guia. - Adios Ngangulero, brisa que el viento me lleva Ague.
Coro. - Brisa que el viento me lleva Ague.
Brisa que el viento me lleva Ague.
Guia. - Adios Ngangulero, brisa que el viento me lleva Ague.
Coro. - Brisa que el viento me lleva Ague.
Brisa que el viento me lleva Ague.
Guia. - Adios Ngangulero, brisa que el viento me lleva Ague.
Coro. - Brisa que el viento me lleva Ague.
Brisa que el viento me lleva Ague.
Guia. - Adios Ngangulero, brisa que el viento me lleva Ague.
Coro. - Brisa que el viento. me lleva Ague.
Brisa que el viento me lleva Ague.
Guia. - Adios Ngarigulero, brisa que el viento me lleva Ague.
Coro. - Brlsa que el viento me lleva Ague.
Brisa que el viento me lleva Ague.
Guia. - Adios Ngatigulero, brisa que el viento me lleva Ague.
Coro. - Brisa que el viento me lleva Ague.
Brisa que el viento me lleva Ague.
Guia. - Adios Ngangulero, brisa que el viento me lleva Ague.
Coro. - Brisa que el viento me lleva Ague.
Brisa que el viento me lleva Ague.
Guia. - Adios Ngangulero, brisa que el vieato me lleva Ague.
Coro. - Brisa que el viento me lleva Ague.
Brisa que el viento me lleva Ague.
Guia. - Adios Ngangulero, brisa que el viento me lleva Ague.
Coro. - Brisa que el viento me lleva Ague.
Brisa que el viento me lleva Ague.
Guia. - Adios Ngangulero, brisa que el viento me lleva Ague.
Coro. - Brisa que el viento me lleva Ague.
Brisa que el viento me lleva Ague.
Guia. - Adios Ngangulero, brisa que el viento me lleva Ague.
Coro. - Brisa que el viento me lleva Ague.
Brisa que el viento me lleva Ague.
Guia. - Adios Ngangulero, brisa que el viento me lleva Ague,
Coro. - Brisa que el viento me lleva Ague.
Brisa que el viento me lleva Ague.
Guia. - Mambe
Coro. - Dias
Guia. - Mambe

"PALO - MAYIMBE"

Coro. - Palo Mayimbe, me llevan pa la Loma.
Guia. - Me llevan pa la Loma, me llevan pa la Loma.
Coro. - Palo Mayimbe, me llevan pa la Loma.
Guia. - Yo corro pa la Loma, yo corro pa la Loma.
Coro. - Palo Mayimbe, me llevan pa la Loma.
Gula. - Yo sube pa la Loma, yo sube pa la Loma.
Coro. - Palo Mayimbe, me llevan pa la Loma.
Guia. - Yo soy 7 Rayos, me llevan pa la Loma.
Coro. - Palo Mayimbe, me llevan pa la Loma.
Guia. - Yo soy Tiembla Terra, me llevan pa la Loma.
Coro. - Palo Mayimbe, me llevan pa la Loma.
Guia. - Yo soy Sholán Guengue, me llevan pa la Loma.
Coro. - Palo Mayimbe, me llevan pa la Loma.
Guia. - Yo soy Madre de Agua, me llevan pa la Loma.
Coro. - Palo Mayimbe, me llevan pa la Loma.
Guia. - Yo sube pa la Loma, yo sube pa la Loma.
Coro. - Palo Mayimbe, me llevan pa la Loma.
Gula. - Yo soy Pata en Llaga, me llevan pa la Loma.
Coro. - Palo Mayimbe, me llevan pa la Loma.
Guia. - Yo soy Centellita, me llevan pa la Loma.
Coro. - Palo Mayimbe, me llevan pa la Loma.
Gula. - Yo soy Lucerito, me llevan pa la Loma.
Coro. - Palo Mayimbe, me llevan pa la Loma.
Gula. - Yo sube pa la Loma, yo sube pa la Loma.
Coro. - Palo Mayimbe, me llevan pa la Loma.
Guia. - Yo sube pa la Loma, yo sube pa la Loma.
Coro. - Palo Mayimbe, me llevan pa la Loma.
Guia. - Mambe.
Coro - Dios.
Guia. - Mambe.
Coro - Dios.
Guia. - Mambe.
Coro - Dios.

"YO SUBE PA LA LOMA"

Yo sube pá la loma, yo sube pá la loma,
Jala y jala, yo jala garabato,
Yo jala garabato, yo jala garabato,
Jala y jala, yo jala garabato,
Yo baja de la loma, yo baja de la loma,
Jala y jala, yo jala garabato,
Y corro pá la loma, yo corro pá la loma,
Jala y jala, yo jala garabato,
Buscando el fundamento, buscando el fundamento,
Jala y jala, yo jala garabato,
Buscando la kinyumba, buscando la kinyumba,
Jala y jala, yo jala garabato,
Buscando mi palo, buscando mi palo,
Jala y jala, yo jala garabato,
Buscando a mi padrino, buscando a mi padrino,
Jala y jala, yo jala garabato,
Buscando a Viento en Ceiba, buscando a Viento en Ceiba,
Jala y jala, yo jala garabato,
Buscando a Mala Fama, buscando a Mala Fama,
Jala y jala, yo jala garabato,
Buscando a 7 Rayos, buscando a 7 Rayos,
Jala y jala, yo jala garabato,
Buscando a Tiembla Tierra, buscando a Tiembla Tierra,
Jala y jala, yo jala garabato,
Buscando a Madre de Agua, buscando a Madre de Agua,
Jala y jala, yo jala garabato,
Buscando a Sholán Guengue, buscando a Sholán Guengue,
Jala y jala, yo jala garabato,
Buscando a la Cuadrilla, buscando a la cuadrilla,
Jala y jala, yo jala garabato,
Buscando al Mayordomo, buscando al Mayordomo,
Jala y jala, yo jala garabato,
Buscando a tó lo empaca, buscando a tó lo empacas,
Jala y jala, yo jala garabato,
Buscando a Manzanero, buscando a manzanero,
Jala y jala, yo jala garabato,
Yo jala garabato, yo jala garabato,
Jala y jala, yo jala garabato,
Buscando a Lucerito, buscando a Lucerito,
Mambe (Dios) Mambe (Dios) Mambe (Dios).

"MAQUINITA"

Coro. - Lligui Llgui Máquina Vapo
Guia. - Son las hora
Coro. - Lligui Llgui Máquina Vapo
Guia. - Jura Menga
Coro. - Lligui Llgui Máquina Vapo
Guia. - Jura Empaca
Coro. - Lligui Llgui Máquina Vapo
Guia. - Jura en Palo
Coro. - Lligui Llgui Máquina Vapo
Guia. - Jura en Fumbi
Coro. - Lligui Llgui Máquina Vapo
Guia. - Maquinita
Coro. - Lligui Llgui Máquina Vapo
Guia. - Jura Enbele
Coro. - Lligui Llgui Máquina Vapo
Guia. - Lucecita.
Coro. - Lligui Llgui Máquina Vapo
Guia. - Jura en Nganga
Coro. - Lligui Lligui Máquina Vapo
Guia. - Maquinita.
Coro. - Lligui Lligui Máquina Vapo
Guia. - Jura en Kisa
Coro. - Lligui Llgui Máquina Vapo
Guia. - Jura Menga
Coro. - Lligui Llgui Máquina Vapo
Guia. - Mambe.
Coro. - Dios.
Guia. - Mambe.
Coro. - Dios.
Gula. - Mambe.
Coro. - Dios.

CHAPTER 10

PALO MONTE VOCABULARY

The language called "Congo" in Cuba derives mostly from KiKongo, a tribal language still spoken in both Congos in Africa as well as in parts of Angola. What follows is the Palo alphabet and a glossary of popular terms employed in the practice of Palo Monte. Where I know the Lukumi, I've also added it to the lexicon. -*Raul Canizares*

THE PALO ALPHABET

A. *yugo*

B. *yulo*

C. *yili*

D. *salvari*

E. *buo*

F. *came*

G. *nie*

H. *busili*

I. *tituli*

J. *yaluni*

K. *tolada*

L. *bi*

M. *duli* (×J

N. *suli* Ɛ×)

Ñ. *bulu* 0•X•0

O. *bisula* ▬

P. *dilonia* ɔ ɔ

Q. *simbula* Ƨx

R. *yolito* (•)

S. *yuriko* ✦/•

T. *bolva* ∅∅

U/V. *soyke* X

W. *sume* V↑X/

X. *saulau* ⊗

Y. *teuse* ✶∿

Z. *kintoo* JIL

GLOSSARY

ENGLISH	CONGO	LUKUMI
	A	
abdomen	nonaloza	ikún
Africa	Juankita	Afrika
aguardiente	malafo	oti
alcohol	malafo-fuaya	
arm (right)	guamono	lembem
ashes	koroa	bebe ina

ENGLISH	CONGO	LUKUMI

B

bag (small)	akuto	wú
beer	malafo-shola	oti agbado
believer	bobbo-keleno	onigbàgbó
bell	egunda	agogo
bird	diendo	eiye
black	nkueto, bufiota	dúdu
body	nkombo	ara
bone	kangome	egungun
bottle	ntumbo	ìgo
bread	kalua	akàrà
bull	nyirango	ako màlû
bush	nfinda	igbo
buttocks	mundana	idi

C

candle	nkinda	ataná
cannon	matonde	ibon nlá
cat	kano-musuako	ológbò
cauldron (empty)	kindeno	ikokó nla
cemetery	campo-afinda, kunasinda	ibi isinkú, ilé, yansan
child	muana	omo
church	munanzo-Zambia	ile-olorun
cigar	nsunga	ashá
cleansing	nsala	ebb
cocodrile	enkumbe-lango	alegba
coconut	canya-emputa	obi
come	kuisa	sunmodo
cooking pot	ikoko	ikoko
crab	agala	akan
cricket	checherengoma	edolo

D

darkness	tombe	su
death	nfuiri	ikú
deity	nkisi	orisha
Devil	Gongoro	Alosi
diviner	nasako	awo
dog	bua, mbwa	ajá
donkey	ceregoa	kétekéte
duck	yanlula	kuekueye

E

earth	ntolo	aiyé
eat	uria	uddia
elephant	tere-nene	ayanakú
enter	kota	wo
evil	ndoki	buruku
evildoer	alembo, nkisi	alaú

F

fan	filé-filé	abebé
father	ntunde, tata	baba
fly (insect)	buanshá	esinsin
friend	bakundi	oluku

G

go	kuenda	lo
God	Zambia	Olodumare
goddaughter	emborayaya	omobinrin orisha
godfather	ndoyeke, tata	babalorisha
godmother	entua, yayi	iyalorisha
godson	emabró	omorisha
good	mbote	rere
guinea-fowl	nsunga-kuda	etú
gunpowder	fula	ekún

H

hat	yerikuame	aketè
hawk	sinfuembo	àwodi
head	lucena	ori
healer	nganga-mune	okoga
heaven	nsulu	orun
hen	yenfelefe	adie
homosexual man	wari-wari	adodí
honey	bonke	onyi
horn (animal)	npake	abani
house	munanzo	ilé
husband	matroko, acar	oko

I

insane	wire-wire	ashiwere
incense	maba guindungo	mu-binu

J

jail	nso-zarabanda	awon
justice	nfumanbata	otito
jutia (Cuban rodent)	egunse-munanzo	akute

K

kill	vonda	pa
king	iyamba, ntinu	oba
kneel	fukama	kunle
knife	embelekoto	obe, pinaldo

L

letter	panda	leta
life	mojo	wiwa laye
lightning	mbandanu	manamana
lion	numa	kiniun
lizard	diansela	alamú

M

machete	embele	adá
man	makala	enia, okunrin
mirror	talatala	awoji
money	nsimio	owó
moon	agonda, mposi	oshu
morning	maksimeni	owúrò
mother	marikiya	iyá
mountain	mongo	oke
mouth	munama	enu

N

necklace	coyera	eleke
nose	nasuro	imú

O

owl	sunsundaka	owiwi

P

parrot	nkore	odide
peanut	nkia	
pheasant	chechewenbala	eyebi agbe, ati aluko
physician	cochino-radau	ologun
pigeon	yenkefo	eiyele
power	lendo, mpati, patti	ashe
pray	dodukila	gbadura
prostitute	ndunga-nsame	panchagara

R

rain	mfula	ojo
rainbow	huyon-guerra	oshumare
razor blade	gele-samba	abe ifari
red	mbuaki	pon

rice	loso	sinkafa
river water	lanso-ganswa	omilodo
rooster	nsuso	akukó
roots	nfitoto	gbongbo

S

sea	mbu	okun
seawater	lanso-kalunga	omilokun
serpent	yoka	eyioko
sheep	nkonde	abo
sickness	yari-yari	arun
skull	kiyumba, kuniako	agbari
song	mambo	suyere
soul	katukemba, nfumbi	emi
speak	vova	wi
spell	bilongo	ogun
star	tenteguia	irawo
stone	matari	otan
street	kiaya	ona
sun	ntangu	orun
sweet potato	bala	batata

T

temple	munanzo, estamfele	igbodu
thanks	entondele	adupe
thunder	mbandanu	ara
tiger	ngo	amotekun
toad	shupa	opolo
today	awe	
tongue	irime	ahon, ede
tooth	enhuto	ehin
tree	nkuni	igi
turkey	ensu-asowa	tolotolo
tying spell	nkangue	linga

133

V

vulture	mayimbe	kole

W

waist	nkuete	ibadi
water	lanso, masa	omi
white (color)	ojibo, mpembe	funfun
white (person)	mundele	
wine	sua, alee	
wind	asolo, kunafinda, mpefe	afefe
woman	ndunka, nkento	obini

Y

yes	inga	en
young	matoco-nkueye	somode

Z

zebra	donko-ceregoa	kétekéte abila

A few useful phrases

Kiambote!: hello! *Wena mafimpi?:* Are you well?
Inga, ye ngeie?: Yes, and you? *fioti ka-ka:* Ah, so-so.
Nkumbu aku inani?: What is your name?
Nkumbu ame i Lumumba: My name is Lumumba
Nsala kiambote: stay well *Nwenda kiambote:* go well
Quien kuenda?: Who goes there?
Somo o no somo! Are we paleros!?
Somo! We are!
Zambia arriba, Zambia abajo, Zambia en to cuatro cotao:
God above, God below, God in all four sides.

APPENDIX 1

After finishing the main text of this book, while working on a future project, a comprehensive study of how herbs are used in Palo and Santeria, I discovered that I had accumulated a number of Spanish-to-English translations of sticks, herbs, and plants that had not been available when I initially wrote the Palo book. Because of the importance of this information for the English-speaking reader, I am including a glossary of such words with their English, Lukumi, and Palo (KiKongo), equivalents as an appendix. With over 200 entries, this may be the largest lexicon of its kind in print. Hopefully, this information will be received with joy by my readers, as many of these translations are not available anywhere else.

SPANISH	LATIN	ENGLISH	LUKUMI	PALO
Abrojo	Tribulus cistides, Lin.	Jamaican Fever plant	Beri Ogun	Fugwe
Acacia	Gliricidia Sepium, Kuth.	Acacia	Sidee	Topia
Achicoria	Leptilon pusillum	Chicory	Amuyo	?
Achiote	Sloanea curatellifolia	Annatto	Baba lye	?
Adormidera	?	Ground tamarind	Erunkumi	?
Aguacate	Persea gratissima	Avocado	Itobi	Akun
Agracejo	Gossypiospermun eriophorus	Bayberry	Yan	Douki
Aguinaldo blanco	Rivea corymbosa	Snake plant	Ewe bere	Tuanso
Aji chile	Capsicum annum	Chili pepper	Cayueddin	Kualau
Aji dulce	Capsicum	Green pepper	Guaro	Mowongo
Aji guaguau	Capsicum baccatum	Hot pepper	Guaguao	Yumbe
Ajonjoli	Sesamun indicum	Sesame	Amati	Ndeba
Alacrancillo	Heliotropium indicum	Indian Heliotrope	Agueyi	Biwoto
Alamo	Ficus religiosa	Peepal	Ofa	Manlofo
Albahaca	Osimun basilicum	Basil	Ororo	Mechuso
Albahaca cimarrona	O. sanctum	Tulasi, Holy basil	Ororo	Mechuso

SPANISH	LATIN	ENGLISH	LUKUMI	PALO
Alcanfor	Cinnamomun camphora	Camphor	Teemi	Gougoro
Algarrobo	Ceratonia siliqua	Carob	Afoma	Flecheo
Algarrobo de olor	Leguminosa mimosoidea	Women's tongue	Ayinre	?
Alga Marina	Fucus Vesiculosus	Kelp	Ewe Okun	?
Algodon	Gossypium arborum	Cotton	Oru	Nduambo
Almacigo	Elaphrium simaruba	Gumbolimbo	Igi Addama	Imbi Iye
Almendro	Terminalis catappa	Almond tree	Iggi ure	Tuanso
Altea	Hibiscus syriacus	Marshmallow	Lukuari	?
Amansa guapo	Chelone glabra	Balmony	Kunino	?
Anamu	Petiveria allicea	Garlic-scented petiveria	Yena	?
Anis	Pinpinella anisum	Anise	Ewe isi	?
Anon	Ammona squamosa	Sweetsop	Irabiri	?
Anil	Idigofera sulfruticosa	Indigo	Yiniya	Firio
Apasote	Chenopodium ambrosioides	Wormseed	Oline	Kosiku
Arbol del cuerno	Acacia cornigera	Bull horn acacia	Maeri	Kwangango
Arbol del sebo	Stillingia sebifera	Florida aspen	Saindi	Kouso
Arroz	Oriza sativa	Rice	Ewo	Loso
Ateje	Cordia collococca	Manjack	Lacheo	Lagwe
Azafran	Carthamus tinctorius	Saffron	Ewe pupo	Mayanda
Azucena	Polianthes tuberosa	Tropical lily	Ododo fun	Torje
Baria	Cordia gerascanthus	Barillo	?	?
Baston de San Francisco	Leonotia nepetaefolia	Lion's ears	Moboro	Tongo
Bejuco de fideos	Cuscuta americana	American dodder	Lobe	?
Bledo	Amaranthus viridis	Slender amaranth	Lobe	?
Boniato	Edulis, Choisy	Sweet potato	Umdukumduku	Mbala
Boton de oro	Spilanthus oleraceus	Golden rod	?	?

SPANISH	LATIN	ENGLISH	LUKUMI	PALO
Caimitillo	Chrysophylum oliviforme	Satin leaf	Didere	?
Caimito	Chrysophylum cainito	Star apple	Asan	Ennua
Caisimon	Piper umbellatum	Umbelate Ig	Iguedi ekuana	Tagwan
Calabaza	Curcubita maxima	Pumpkin	Eleguedde	Male
Campana	Datura stramonium	Thorn apple	Agogo	Kusuambo
Canela del monte	Canella wonterana	Wild cinnamon	Dedi	Mokocagwando
Canutillo	Comelina elegans	Scouring rush	Ewe karodo	Totoi
Cana de azucar	Saccharum offinarum	Sugar cane	Igguere	Musenga
Caña brava	Bambusa vulgaris	Bamboo	Pako	Endosongo
Caña fistula	Cassia fistula	Purging cassia	Ifefe	?
Caña hueca	Arundo dorax	redgrass	Ifefe	?
Cañamazo amargo	Paspalum conjugatum	Hilo grass	Ogbo	?
Cañamazo dulce	Azonopus compressus	Centipede grass	Ogbo	?
Caoba	Swietenia mahogani	Mahogany	Ayan	Yuknia
Cardo santo	Argemone mexicana	Mexican poppy	Ika	Cando ere
Cebolla	Allium cepa	Onion	Alubosa	Tenje-tenje
Cedro	Cedrela mexicana	Cedar 01	Opepe	Nkunia menga
Chirimoya	Anona reticulate	Netted custard apple	Mequeri	Biloko
Cipres	Cupressus funebris	Cypriss	Iggiku	Sambiantuka
Ciruela	Spondias cironella	Plum	Iggi Yeye	?
Clavos de olor	Eugenia caryphylla	Cloves	?	?
Coco	Cocos ncifera	Coconut	Obi	Sandu
Copey	Clusia rosea	Autograph tree	Inlanna	?
Coquito africano	Cola acuminata	Kola nut	Obi Kola	?
Corjo	Acreemia crispa Amyris	Palm	Epo	Gesi
Cuaba	Balsamifera	Weat Indian Rosewood	Loaso	Inkita
Cucaracha	Zebrina pendula	Wandering Jew	Añal	Kienguene
Culantro	Coriandrum sativum	Coriander	Ichop	Bianki

SPANISH	LATIN	ENGLISH	LUKUMI	PALO
Daguilla	Logetta linteares	Lace bark tree	?	?
Escoba amarga	Pdarthenium hysterophore	Cut-leaved Parthenium	Eggweniye	Baombo
Espinaca	Spinacea oleracea	Spinach	Obado	Mbi mbi
Estropajo	Luffa luffa	Loofa	?	?
Eucalypto	Eucalyptus globulos	Eucalyptus	?	?
Flor de Aqua	Eichornia azurea	Rooted water hyacinth	Ayuoro	Irituu
Flor de Mayo	Laelia ancepa	Purple orchid	Weginu	?
Flor de muerto	Calendula officinalis	Marigold	?	?
Framboyan	Delonix regla	Royal poinciana	Iggi tambina	?
Fruta bomba	Carica papaya	Papaya	Idefe	Machafio
Galan de dia	Cestrum diurum	Day-blooming Jasmine	Orufirin	Dondoko
Galan de noche	Cestrum nocturnum	Night-blooming Jasmine	Orufirin	Montoo
Gandul	Cajanus indicus	Pidgeon pea	?	?
Genciana de la tierra	Voyra aphylla	Gentian	Iyendere	Lonlo
Genjibre	Zingiber officinale	Ginger	Ewe atale	?
Geranio	Pelargonium odorattisimum	Geranium	Pupayo	?
Girasol	Helianthus annuns	Sunflower	Yongoso	?
Grajo	Eugenia axillaria	White stopper	?	?
Grama	Cynadon dactylon	Common grass	Ewe eran	Guandi
Grama de cabakko	?	Goose grass	?	?
Granada	Punica granatum	Pomegranate	Oroco	?
Guacamaya amarilla	Poinciana pulcherrima	Yellow poinciana	Orumaya	?

SPANISH	LATIN	ENGLISH	LUKUMI	PALO
Guaco	Aristolochia serpentaria	Virginia snake root	?	?
Guacumo	?	Guazuma tree	?	?
Guanabana	Anona muricata	Soursop	Iggi omo fun	Ombandinga
Guanina	Senna occidentalis	Stinking weed	Kropomu	?
Guano	Copernica glabrescens	Straw	Mariwo	Molunse
Guira	Crescentia cujete	Narrow - leaved calabash	?	?
Guayacan	Guayacum offinalis	Lignum vitae tree	?	Yunkagwa
Guayaba	Psidium guajaba	Guava	Kenku	Guankibilunga
Helcho de rio	Osmunda regalis	River fern	?	?
Henequen	Agave americana	Maguey	Kunweko	?
Hicaco	Chrysobalanus icaco	Green coco plum	Kinseke	Mungaoko
Higuera	Fecus carica	Fig	Poto	?
Higuereta	Ricinus comunes	Castor	?	?
Hinojo	Foeniculum vulgare	Fennel	Koriko	?
Huevo de gallo	Tabernaemontana vulgare	Dog bane	?	?
Incienso	Artemisa abrotatum	Southernwood	Turare	?
Itamo real	?	Slipper plant	?	?
Jaboncillo	Spinadus saponaria	Common soap berry	Obueno	Langui
	Genupa americana	Marmalade Box tree	?	?
Jagua			?	Goontongo
Jobo	Spedias membin		Abba	Grengerenge

SPANISH	LATIN	ENGLISH	LUKUMI	PALO
Lampazo	Arctium lappa	Burdock	?	?
Laurel	Ficus nitida	Bay laurel	Iggi nile	Ocereke
Lechuga	Lactuca sativa	Lettuce	Ilenke	?
Lengua de vaca	Rumex obtusifolius	Yellow dock	?	?
Limo de mar	?	Seaweed	Ewe Olokun	?
Limon	Citrus limonum	Lemon	Oroko	Koronko
Lirio	Lilium	Lily	Merefe	Tunkanso
Llamoa	?	Muskwood	?	?
Llanten	Plantago lanceolata	Ribwort plantain	Chechere	?
Macio	Typha rhomboidea	Cat tail	Ewe egun	?
Madreselva	Lonicera spp.	Honey suckle	?	?
Majagua	Parititi tiliaceum	Mountain mahoe	?	Musenguene
Maiz	zea maya	corn	Ikeri	?
Malacara	Plumbago scandens	Blue colored lead wort	Mubino	?
Malanga	Xantosoma sagitfolium	Dasheen	Ikoku	Nkumbia
Malanguita	?	Japanese potato	?	?
Malva blanca	?	Ceasar weed	Dede Fun	Dubue
Mango	Mangifera indica	mango	Oro	Ema benga
Mani	Arachis hypogaca	Peanut	Epa	Mindo
Manzanilla	Cythanthellum americanum	Chamomile	Nikirio	Dumbuande
Marañon	Anacardium occidentale	Cashew	?	?
Maravilla	Mirabilis jalapa	Common marvel of Peru	Ewe ewa	Boddule
Mastuerzo	Lepidium virginicum	Virginia pepper grass	Eribo	?
Mejorana	Origanum marjoram	Marjarum	?	?
Melon de agua	Citrullus citrulla	Watermelon	Agbeye	Machafio
Melon de castilla	Cucumis melo	Cantaloupe	Eggure	Machafio

SPANISH	LATIN	ENGLISH	LUKUMI	PALO
Mife	Eugenio rhombea	Red stopper	?	?
Millo	Hulcus sorghum	Millet	?	?
Mirto	Murraya exotica	Myrtle	Urari	?
Naranjo	Citrus auratum	Orange tree	Orolocun	Maamba
Naranjo agria	Citrus bigardia	Sour orange	Korosan	?
Ñame	Dioscorea alata	African yam	Iyerosun	Loato
Ojo de buey	Mucuna urens	Velvet bean	Jumiyi	?
Ojo de raton	Rivina humiles	Pony's foot	Moddobo	?
Orozuz de la tierra	Lippia dulcis	Aztec sweet herb	Eyefoo	Inmeyemo
Palo dulce	Glycyrrhiza glabra	Licorice	?	?
Palo yaya	Oxandra lanceolata	Black lancewood	Denkuyero	?
Pendejera	Solanum torvum	Turkey berry	Isiami	Milisia
Peonia	Abrus pecatorius	Peony, Crab eyes	Ewereyeye	?
Perejil	Apium petroselinum	Parsley	Isako	Ntuoro
Pica pica	Stizolobium pruriens	Cow itch	Sisi	Ote
Pimienta	piper nigrum	Black pepper	Ata	Esakukaku
Pino	pinus tropicalis	Pine	Okilan	Bundumoye
Piñon botija	Curcas curcas	Physic nut	Addo	Puluka
Pitahaya	Cactus pitaiaya	Pitajala	Esogi	Belongo
Platano	Musa paradisiaca	Plaintain	Oguede	Makondo
Pringa hermosa	Tragia voluble	Twining tragia	Okorere	Nkato
Prodigiosa	Kalanchoe piinnata	Life everlasting	?	?

SPANISH	LATIN	ENGLISH	LUKUMI	PALO
Quimbombo	Hibiscus esculentus	Okra	Alila	Gondei
Rabo de zorra	Igitaria insularis	Silk grass	?	?
Reseda	Lawsonia inermis	Henna	?	?
Romerillo	Bidens alba	Shepherd's needle	?	?
Rompe saraguey	Eupatorium odoratum	Boneset	Tabate	Ntema
Ruda	ruta graveolens	Rue	Atopa kun	?
Ruibarbo	?	Rhubarb	Eruko ewe kan	?
Sabila	Aloe vera	Aloe vera	?	?
Salvadera	Hara crepitans	Sandbox tree	Aronica	?
Salvia de castilla	Salvia officinalis	Sage	Kiriwi	Vitti leka
Sanguinaria	?	Blood root	?	?
Sauco	?	Willow	?	?
Sauco blanco	?	American elder	?	?
Siempreviva			?	
San Diego	Gomphrena globosa	Globe amaranth	Ayarayere	?
Sargazo	Sargassum vulgares	Seaweed	?	?
Sasafras	Sassafras varifolium	Sassafras	Eran kumi	?
Sensitiva	Acacia dealbata	Mimosa	Atori	?
Siguaraya	Trichilla havanensis	Bastard lime		Inso

SPANISH	LATIN	ENGLISH	LUKUMI	PALO
Tartago	?	Physic nut	?	?
Tabaco	Nicotiana tabacum	Tabacco	Ewe etaba	Nsunga
Tamarindo	Tamarindus indica	Tamarind	Iggi iyagbon	?
Toronjil	Melissa officinalis	Lemon balm	Ewe tuni	?
Tomate	Lycopersicum esculentum	Tomato	Ichoma	Korogondo
Trebol	Trifolium repens	Shamrock	Ewe etameri	Kanda
Tuna	Euphorbia lactea	Cactus	Weggun	?
Uña de gato	Momisia iguanale	Cat's claw	?	?
				?
Vacabuey	Curatilla americana	Sandpaper tree	?	?
Vainilla	Epidendrum vainilla	Vanilla	?	?
Verbena	Verbena officinalis	Vervain	Orrioyo	?
Verdulaga	Tanilum paniculatum (see sensitiva)	Purslane	?	?
Vergonzosa				
Vicaria	Vinca rosea	Periwinkle	?	?
Violeta	Violeta odorata	African violet	Luko	?
Yamao	Guarea guidonia	Muskwood	Fendebillo	Nkita
Yerba buena	Mentha sativa	Mint	Efirin	?
Yerba fina	?	Lawn grass	?	?
Yerba mora	Solanum americanum	Pop bush	?	?
Yerba de sangre	?	Butterfly sage	?	?
Zarzaparilla	?	Sasparilla	?	?

APPENDIX II:
ACTA CIFRADA, AN ACTUAL INITIATION NOTEBOOK.

Much has been written about the fabled "libretas" (notebooks) that Paleros receive when they become initiated. What do these notebooks look like? Here we reproduce one of these libretas, giving also an English translation of its contents.

Translation

Page 1 Written account:
Today, June 12, 1995 in the city of New York, in the House of Tiembla Tierra Camposanto Medinoche Bien Plantao, Narayan Ramos was initiated as Tata Nkisi, having undergone all the ceremonies of our Religion with the blessings of the Guardian Spirits.
Hia iniating Tata was: Camposanto Medianoche
House Godmother: Yayi Balunde
Witnesses: Acheró, Juan Valdes (Tata Mingo), Karl Ortiz, Eddie Barnett and Nkoto Sandi .

y damos reconocimiento
y se' los arriba firmantes,
con la ayuda de sombra.
Al pino nuevo Narayan
Ramos se juró por: Centella
Ndoki.
su papá es: Lucero Viramundo
lo alumbró: Eddie Barnett

Palo que come con su Cabeza: ~~~~
Guara.

su nombre: Nsambi Kienvence
Hasta que Nfuiri (6.12.95)

Translation

We the above signers hereby testify to the veracity of these proceedings
with the aid of the guardian spirits. The neophyte Narayan Ramos was,
sworn under: Centella Ndoki,
his father being: Lucero Viramundo,
his sponsor: Eddie Barnett,
stick that eats with his head: Guara,
his name: Nsambi Kienvence,
hasta que Nfuiri (6/12/95)

(3)

Registro de los 7 dias

Tiene que limpiarce ante
Sucero Todas las Semanas

Le Salén grandes TRiunfos
musicales

Habla de pasar + nabajos
un Tiempo, pero despues
Tendra mucho dinero.
tiene que recibir 7 rayos
tiene que recibir
Sucero mundo para
firmeza en el muerto

tabús: no comer manzanas
rojas, no comer arijoles
blancos.

Se le hizo registro de los
7 dias

Translation

Has to be cleansed in front of Lucero every week.
Great musical triumphs will come to him.
Speaks of undergoing hardships for awhile, but later having much money.
Has to receive Siete Rayos.
Has to receive Lucero Mundo for firmness with the dead.
Taboos: Cannot eat red apples or white beans.
So ends the seven day reading.

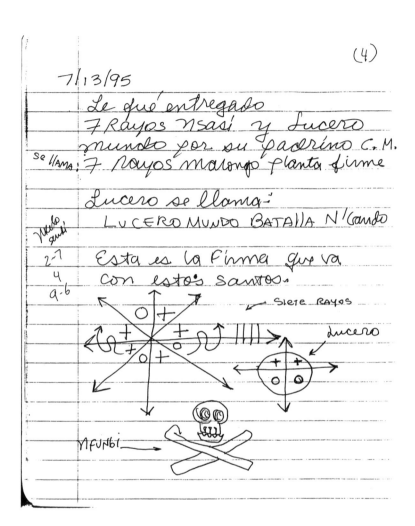

7/13/95

Le qué entregado
7 Rayos Nsasi y Lucero
mundo por su padríno C.M.
se llama: 7 Rayos Malongo planta firme

Lucero se llama:
LUCERO MUNDO BATALLA N'Gando

Esta es la Firma que va
con estos santos.

SIETE RAYOS

Lucero

Nfumbi

Translation

7/13/95
Has received Siete Rayos Nsasi and Lucero Mundo this day by the hand of his Godfather C.M.
Name of his deity: Siete Rayos Malongo Planta Firme
Name of his Lucero: Lucer Mundo Batalla N'Gando. This is the Sygill that goes with these Deities.

(5)

Registro que mando
a hacer 7 rayos.

Abrió con Zarabanda Ellife
madre de agua. Ellife

7 Rayos itagua alafia

Grandes · cambios en su
vidas; peleas con el
padrino pero se resolveran
tiene que aprender todos
los secretos, pues esta
destinado a ser un
gran rey y un Famoso
artista.
Puede hacer brujerías y
trabajar con lo malo —
— Ellife —

Nkobo
4
6-6-4
6-4

Translation

Reading ordered by Seite Rayos:
Opened with Zarabando Eyife
Madre de Agua Eyife
Seite Rayos Itagua Alafia
Great changes in your life ,
fights with your Godfather, but will end in peace.
You must learn all secrets for you are destined to be a great king and a famous artist.
The way to dark magic is open to you.   -Eyife

BIBLIOGRAPHY

Bolivar Arostegui et al: *Los Orishas en Cuba,* Ediciones Union, Havana, Cuba, 1990.

_____ :   *Ta Makuende Yaya y las reglas de Palo Monte,* Ediciones Union: Havana, Cuba, 1998.

Cabrera, Lydia: *El Monte,* Ediciones Universal, Miami, 1986.

_____ :   *La Regla Kimbisa del Santo Cristo del Buen Viaje,* Peninsula Printing Inc., Miami, 1977.

_____ :   *Las Reglas de Congo:* Palo Monte, Mayombe, Coleccion del Chichereku en el Exilic, Miami, 1979.

Farris Thompson, Robert: *Flash of the Spirit,* Random House, New York, 1984.

Gomez, Demetrio: *Various unpublished, undated, notebooks* c. 1889-1925.

Numerous firmas (sigils) were collected in situ at the homes and temples of many paleros.

The author, Baba Raul Canizares, Tata Camposanto Medianoche, also relied on literally thousands of pages of field notes of interviews with over 200 practitioners over a span of twenty years and on his own libretas and those of many others who selflessly allowed him ample access to their treasures. At last count these field notes amounted to nearly 8,000 pages. In 1992 the department of Religious Studies at University of South Florida, one of the most distinguished in the world, after careful consideration of Baba Raul's research and the uniqueness and validity of his field notes (after the Carlos Castaneda scandal, they wanted to make sure the field notes were worthy) awarded him a Masters degree in Religious studies, the resulting Masters' thesis has been published in two parts, first as a book concentrating on Santeria, and the second is the present work, the Book on Palo.

ABOUT THE AUTHOR

Respected scholar, award-winning poet and essayist, world-renowned artist, innovative musician: Baba Raul Canizares is truly Santería's renaissance man. His scholarly articles have appeared in numerous journals of opinion, such as Si. Uvgy, A *Journal of Alternative Religions*, as well as in India's *Journal of Dharma*, Jamaica's *Caribbean Quarterly*, and Sri Lanka's *Ethnic Studies Reports*, to name a few. Baba Raul has won the prestigious Enrique Jose Varona literary prize in nearly every category-poetry, short story, and essay. He has addressed national meetings of the American Academy of Religions several times, and has lectured at UCLA in Los Angeles, Colby College in Waterville, Maine, as well as at the Open Center, the Afro-Caribbean Cultural Center, and the Learning Annex in New York City. At University of South Florida Baba Raul designed and taught the first full-credit Santería course ever offered by a major American university. His book *Cuban Santería, Walking with the Night is* considered a classic. Originally published in 1992, an expanded edition appeared in 1999 and has already outsold the first. As a painter and sculptor, Baba's work has been exhibited at such prestigious venues as Cavin-Morris, the leading gallery for Afro-Caribbean folk artists in New York City, and at Baltimore's Folk Art Museum. He has been the subject of three different one-man-shows at Clayton's Gallery in Manhattan's Lower East Side. Art critic Luis Perez, writing for *El Espectador* in Puerto Rico, called Baba's Eleggua figures "some of the most important sculptures of the latter part of the twentieth century." Baba has also received acclaim as a cover artist and illustrator for his own books as well as those of others. He is also a cartoonist. Biblical scholar Dr. James Strange, at the time Chair of University of South Florida's Religious Studies Department, wrote this about Baba: "Simply put, Raul is the most distinguished M.A. student we have graduated in the nearly ten year life of this program." A former adjunct professor of Religious Studies at University of South Florida, Baba also holds degrees in Liberal Arts and Psychology. Baba Raul Canizares is the founding oba (spiritual leader) of the Orisha Consciousness Movement, with members worldwide. He lives in New York City, surrounded by loving godchildren who see him as a world teacher and conduit to the Divine Mind.

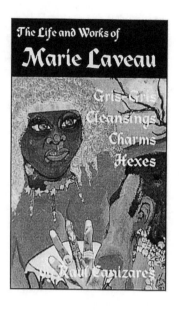

The Life and Works of
Marie Laveau
Gris-Gris, Cleansings, Charms & Hexes
by Raul Canizares

In the early 1800's Marie Laveau at the age of 36, reigned as queen of all Voodoo in New Orleans and the surrounding areas. She made the practice of Voodoo a commercial venture and charged large sums for her services. She attracted customers from every class and creed in search of aid from her supernatural powers.

Marie had a great many charms and amulets which she used and guaranteed. All of her magical Voodoo rituals and items were said to achieve the desired end result. The recipes in this book come directly from Marie's personal notebooks... *perhaps they'll work for you!*

ISBN 0-942272-71-4 5½"x 8½" 66 PAGES $5.95

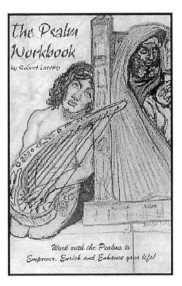

The Psalm Workbook

by Robert Laremy

WORK WITH THE PSALMS TO
EMPOWER, ENRICH AND ENHANCE YOUR LIFE!

This LARGE PRINT King James version of the Book of Psalms contains nearly 400 simple rituals and procedures that can be used to help you accomplish anything you desire. Use the situational index provided to decide which psalm to pray for your specific need.

Peace, Protection, Health,
Success, Money, Love,
Faith, Inspiration, Spiritual Strength
And much more!

Approach your worship with a clean heart and a child-like faith in God's infinite wisdom and you will derive tremendous results from the powers of the psalms.

ISBN 0-942272-68-4 5½"x 8½" 202 pages $7.95

WWW.ORIGINALPUB.COM   Toll Free: 1 (888) OCCULT - 1

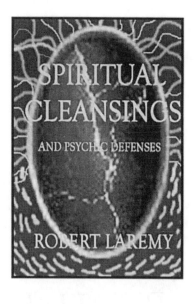

$7.95

SPIRITUAL CLEANSINGS & PSYCHIC DEFENSES

By Robert Laremy

PSYCHIC ATTACKS ARE REAL AND THEIR EFFECTS CAN BE DEVASTATING TO THE VICTIM. NEGATIVE VIBRATIONS CAN BE AS HARMFUL AS BACTERIA, GERMS AND VIRUSES. THERE ARE TIME HONORED METHODS OF FIGHTING THESE INSIDIOUS AND PERNICIOUS AGENTS OF DISTRESS. THESE TECHNIQUES ARE DESCRIBED IN THIS BOOK AND THEY CAN BE APPLIED BY YOU. NO SPECIAL TRAINING OR SUPERNATURAL POWERS ARE NEEDED TO SUCCESSFULLY EMPLOY THESE REMEDIES. ALL OF THE PROCEDURES DESCRIBED IN THIS BOOK ARE SAFE AND EFFECTIVE, FOLLOW THE INSTRUCTIONS WITHOUT THE SLIGHTEST DEVIATION. THE CLEANSINGS PROVIDED ARE INTENDED AS ""*OVER THE COUNTER*" *PRESCRIPTIONS* TO BE USED BY ANYONE BEING VICTIMIZED BY THESE AGENTS OF CHAOS.

ISBN 0-942272-72-2 5½"x 8½" 112 pages $7.95

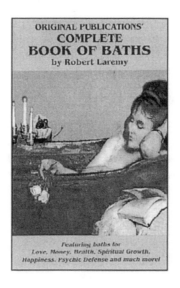

Original Publications Complete Book of Baths

BY ROBERT LAREMY

**FEATURING RECIPES FOR
LOVE, MONEY, HEALTH,
HAPPINESS, SPIRITUAL GROWTH,
PSYCHIC DEFENSE,
FIGHTING BAD HABITS
AND MUCH MORE!**

ISBN 0-942272-73-0 5½"x 8½" 94 pages $6.95